A Message from the Author

Right now, you are holding one of the key factors to you becoming a REAL Nurse

Quick Facts for NCLEX® is by far our best-selling NCLEX® Study Guide and the foundation of the ReMar V2 Program! This study guide is designed to give you Core Content in a simple, easy-to-understand, "no nonsense" structure that will help you quickly identify your strengths and analyze areas of weakness. With *Quick Facts*, you will immediately begin to comprehend many of the major areas that are essential to passing NCLEX® RN & PN.

YOUR SUCCESS IN NURSING

Your success in nursing is determined by your ability to think, plan, decide, and take-action These same skills are necessary when preparing to take NCLEX®. The stronger you are with the fundamentals, the faster you will learn how to critically think.

With *Quick Facts* as your primary study guide, you are on the right track to achieve the same types of results as our students who have passed NCLEX® and are now living out their dreams.

Whether you're starting nursing school tomorrow or graduated years ago, I want to encourage you to stay focused on your goals. Let's put pride to the side, cast away doubt, feelings of inadequacy, and anything that does not support this one effort here and now. I have personally beaten the odds and have helped thousands of nurses just like you to do the same.

I've created several resources to help you along this journey including my ReMar Nurse RN & LPN *YouTube Channel, Ultimate Next Gen NCLEX Study Guide, and FREE Trial to the ReMar NCLEX V2 Review for Next Gen – available now at ReMarNurse.com.*

I know that studying for NCLEX can be challenging. My goal is to help you study the content and make this process as simple as possible. If you have any questions as you study, I want you to contact me directly, my email is Support@ReMarReview.com. Stay focused; put faith over fear and continue to invest in yourself because YOU CAN, YOU WILL, and YOU MUST Pass NCLEX!

Regina M. Callion MSN, RN
www.ReMarNurse.com

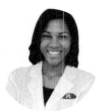

ReMar Nurse RN & LPN

200K subscribers (almost there... but only if you sub ☺)

Subscribe to my YouTube for weekly Reviews!

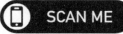
SCAN ME

The ReMar Review Quick Facts for NCLEX®

First Printing, 2010; Revised 2012, 2014, 2015, 2017, 2018, 2019, 2020, 2023

ISBN: 1-7339414-9-5

S.M.C. Medical Media

Ordering Information:

Quantity sales- Special discounts are available on quantity purchases by educational institutions, not-for-profits, corporations, associations, and others. For details, contact the publisher at the address above.

Orders by U.S. & International trade bookstores and wholesalers. Please contact ReMar Review:

Email us: Support@ReMarReview.com or visit www.ReMarNurse.com

*NCLEX, NCLEX-RN, NCLEX-PN are registered trademarks of the National Council of State Boards of Nursing, Inc. (NCSBN). NCSBN is not affiliated with ReMar Review or this educational publication.

Medical Disclaimer: The information contained in this book is intended for educational purposes only and is the opinion of the author. It is not intended to be a substitute for professional and medical advice, diagnosis, or treatment. Always seek the advice of your physician or other qualified healthcare provider with any questions you may have regarding a medical condition. Never disregard professional medical advice or delay in seeking it because of something your read. The author does not recommend or endorse any specific tests, physicians, products, procedures, opinions, or other information mentioned in this book.

$49.95
ISBN 978-1-7339414-9-5
54995>

9 781733 941495

How to use Quick Facts for NCLEX®

Believe me when I tell you that you need to know everything in this book and memorize it from cover to cover! There is no skipping around with *Quick Facts,* everything is essential!

Many of our nurses call Quick Facts their NCLEX Bible because they take it EVERYWHERE they go! Be sure to review this book multiple times before testing as you need to know this content like the back of your hand!

Finally, no matter how much pressure you feel about this test, keep your total study times under three hours each day to avoid mental fatigue and nursing burnout. Your nursing career is too important to cram for. Be consistent with your study times and take one or two days off each week to allow your mind to process what you have learned.

Quick Facts Study Calendar

Week 1				
Monday	Tuesday	Wednesday	Thursday	Friday
QF pages. 1-10		QF pages. 11-20		QF pages. 21-30
QF Pharmacology	QF Pharmacology Only	QF Pharmacology		QF Pharmacology
Allergy Medications Analgesics	Anticonvulsants Antidotes	Cardiac Medications	Review pages 1-20	Cardiac Medications
Antibiotics	Antineoplastics	Hypertension Focused Meds	Reread Challenging	Digoxin Nitroglycerin
Anticoagulants	Anti-Parkinsons		Areas studied	

Week 2				
QF pages. 31-40		QF pages. 41-50	QF pages. 51-60	QF Pharmacology
QF Pharmacology	QF Pharmacology	QF Pharmacology	QF Pharmacology	Benzodiazepines
	GI Medications	Oral Antidiabetics	Maternity	Non-benzodiazepines
Diuretics	Insulins	Natural Alternatives	Respiratory	
				or Review challenging areas

Week 3				
QF pages. 61-70	QF pages. 71-80	QF pgs. 81+	Read Cultural	
QF Pharmacology	QF Pharmacology	QF Pharmacology	Considerations	Scan the code to get
Antidepressants	Anti-Psychotics	TV drugs	Review difficult areas	the FREE Trial of the rest
SSRIs	Atypical Antipsychotics	Quick Pharmacology Sheet	from each week.	of the program. Watch classes, create Next Gen Case Studies
MAOIs	Typical Antipsychotics			

Next Steps for NCLEX!

See page V

ReMar NCLEX Planner Page

As we begin this phase of your nursing journey, I want to welcome you into the ReMar Nurse family. My goal for you is two-fold. First, we'll teach you the fundamental nursing content that you need to know to create a strong foundation for NCLEX.

Beyond the content, my goal is to help you become an amazing nurse with the ability to reach the highest level of our nursing profession. This is nursing, and this is what it means to be a ReMar Nurse.

Name:	Date:

I will pass NCLEX by doing these 4 things:
1. Focusing on the content
2.
3.
4.

Why I need to pass NCLEX:

What are my 3 biggest barriers to studying for NCLEX?

1.
2.
3.

To become more productive, I am willing to sacrifice:

Today I am grateful for:

Take a moment to complete this page as you plan for the journey ahead and the necessary adjustments that you will need to make in order to reach your nursing goals!

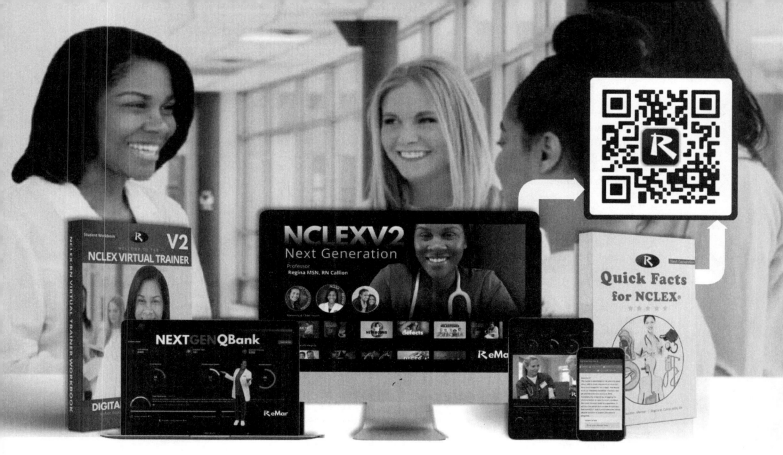

Comprehensive Next Generation NCLEX Prep Course

If you're a nursing student, the NGN can be intimidating. But don't worry! ReMar has your back!

Get easy access to Professor Regina's exclusive **Content Lectures**, **NGN Question Bank**, and **Computer Adaptive Self-Assessment (CAT) exams** to help you ace the Next Generation NCLEX Exam. With ReMar, students are provided with concise core content that will enable you to pass with confidence with our four-week study calendar for the **NCLEX-V2 Program**!

Scan the QR code or go to ReMarNurse.com to complete your NGN CONTENT Lecture training! Yup it's super affordable because our goal is to be a blessing and help the right nurses pass NGN this year. If you want to explore the NCLEX-V2 review, grab your phone, go to the site or scan the code to create an **Unlimited FREE Trial account** with no credit card needed. You can also delay your starting date up to 90 days to lock in today's discount price!

UNDERSTAND NEXT GEN FASTER

V2 - ONE STOP RESOURCE NGN

- Content Lectures
- NGN Question Bank
- CAT Assessments
- Digital Workbook
- Best NGN Professor
- Study in 4 weeks
- 99.2% Student Success*

Complete your training now in just!

30 days or less

Create your Free Trial Account

Join today at ReMarNurse.com

TABLE OF CONTENTS

ABO Blood Groups

What is the ABO antigen system?	It is the different classes of human blood.
What part of the blood is classified?	The red blood cells are distinguished.
What other blood is compatible with Type A?	Type A or O
What other blood is compatible with Type B?	Type B or O
What other blood is compatible with Type O?	Type O + or O -
What other blood is compatible with Type AB?	Type A, B, or O

Clinical Priority	1. Blood transfusions are ordered for clients with hypovolemia caused by hemorrhage, anemia, or blood clotting deficiencies.
	2. A doctor's order is needed for each blood transfusion. 2 licensed nurses must verify before the transfusion starts.
	3. Other types of blood products include: packed red blood cells, platelets, fresh frozen plasma, albumin, clotting factors and cryoprecipitate.

Abortions

Types	Contractions	Bleeding	Cervical Dilatation	Amniotic Sac	Nursing Considerations
Complete	No, the body has expelled all the products of pregnancy (blood, tissue, & embryo).	Yes or no both are possible afterwards.	Closed-because the uterus no longer has the embryo, fetus or placenta.	Unable to detect one.	Monitor mother post-delivery. Provide emotional support.
Incomplete	Yes or no both are possible.	Yes	Open-the baby or parts of placenta may still be present	Ruptured	The mother still needs to pass fetal tissue parts.
Inevitable	Yes	Yes	Open-the baby is no longer able to survive.	Ruptured	Abortion will eventually occur.
Missed	No-this is also called a silent abortion.	Yes, a small amount is expected. However, there may be no pain, cramping, or bleeding at all.	Closed-the body does not detect the fetus has died.	Unable to detect or present.	Monitor the mother. Medical and surgical treatment (vacuum aspiration, misoprostol) are both options for the management of missed abortions.
Threatened	Yes or no both are possible.	Yes or no both are possible.	Closed-the fetus is still inside of the uterus.	Intact	Fetus is still alive. All measures to save fetus should be initiated. A complete bedrest with no bathroom privileges is expected. Monitor mother and fetus.

Acid Reflux (GERD)

What is the primary symptom?	Heartburn (pyrosis)
What test confirms GERD?	Barium swallow fluoroscopy
What body part malfunction occurs in GERD?	The lower esophageal sphincter

Clinical Priority

1. Teach the patient to eat small frequent meals which creates less hydrochloric acid.

2. Patients should remain upright for 30 minutes after every meal.

3. Patients should avoid food items which create more acid such as orange juice or tomatoes.

4. The use of antacids should be encouraged. Antacids should be taken 1 hour before or after other medications. Antacids can also cause constipation.

Acquired Immunodeficiency Syndrome

What is the virus that causes AIDS?	**Human Immunodeficiency Virus (HIV)**
How is HIV transmitted?	Sexual intercourse Direct contact with infected blood or body fluids such as semen and breast milk.
What are the symptoms of HIV?	Fever, weight loss, night sweats, diarrhea, fatigue
How is the presence of HIV confirmed?	Screening is done FIRST to see if the HIV antibodies are present the test is performed to identify the HIV antibodies.
What is the screening test?	ELISA
What is ELISA?	It is the enzyme-linked immunosorbent assay. A blood test that uses special enzymes that attach to blood.
What confirms the screening test?	HIV differentiation assay Western Blot is no longer used.
How does HIV attack the body?	It attacks the immune system by destroying T- lymphocytes. The virus also rapidly self-replicates.
What is so important about T-lymphocytes?	T cells help the immune system to recognize and fight pathogens.

What is another name for T-lymphocytes?

CD4 cells

Why is the CD4 count important?

The lower the CD4 count, the more damage the virus has done to the body.

What is a normal CD4 count in a patient without HIV?

500-1500 in healthy adults.

What is the normal CD4 count in a patient with HIV?

Anything at or above 500 means the patient is in good health. If the CD4 count is below 200, the HIV has progressed to AIDS.

If a patient's CD4 count is below 200, the patient is at risk for what?

Opportunistic infections.

What is a nucleic acid test (NATs)?

This is a test for the viral load of HIV in the blood.

List some opportunistic infections.

-Oral pharyngeal candida infection (mouth fungus)
-Kaposi's sarcoma (skin cancer)
-Pneumocystis pneumonia
-Cytomegalovirus (blindness)
-Meningitis

What is the goal of HIV medications?

To interfere with the virus replicating inside of the patient.

The most important medication to know for NCLEX is _____?

Zidovudine

Which isolation precautions are used with HIV?

Universal precautions.
All blood should be suspected of HIV as patients do not have to tell anyone they have HIV. The nurse should treat blood or body fluid as if it is infected.

How do isolation precautions change with AIDS?

If the patient has a low CD4 count and is at risk of an opportunistic infection:
The patient should have a
-Private room
-Reverse isolation
-RN/PN should wear gloves, gown, goggles, mask when in direct contact with blood or body fluids.

What are the teaching points for parents who have a child with HIV?	- Clean up body fluid/ blood with 10:1 water/ bleach ratio. - The child should get all immunizations, except lives vaccines such as: <u>MMR</u>, <u>varicella</u>, & <u>oral poliovirus.</u> - Feed child a high-calorie & protein diet -Use gloves to change diapers.

Clinical Priority	1. All suspected clients should be tested immediately. 2. The beginning of antiretroviral therapy should be started rapidly. This a major priority. 3. Cognitive behavioral therapy, peer support, and medication compliance are necessary components of positive health care.

Acute Renal Failure

What is the definition of acute renal failure (ARF)?	The sudden loss of kidney function to excrete toxins and regulate fluid and electrolytes
What are some possible causes of ARF?	Infection, obstruction, shock
There are three phases; say what they are?	The oliguric, diuretic, and recovery phase.
During the oliguric phase, what should the nurse expect to see clinically?	This phase lasts 1 to 2 weeks. A low urine output of less than 400 ml per day, hyperkalemia, hypertension, elevated BUN/creatinine levels, and fluid overload.
What two electrolytes will be elevated?	Sodium and phosphate
The diuretic phase is second; what is expected?	The urine output slowly returns, hypokalemia, and hypotension. BUN/creatinine decreases but still elevated.
What does the recovery phase mean?	The kidneys are recovering through a slow process. The GFR increases which allows urine output to increase. The BUN and creatinine return to normal.
Which is the best diet for a client with ARF?	*Healthy carbs, low protein, and low sodium

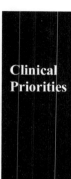

Clinical Priorities

The client will be placed on fluid restrictions. It is appropriate for the *nurse's aide* to hang any educational sign over the bed or inside the room. <u>Never hang patient information signs outside of the room. It is HIPPA violation.</u>

Daily weights are required.

Monitor the patient for azotemia which is the development of urea in the blood.

Monitor the patient's mental status as confusion and lethargy are caused by a buildup of toxins in blood.

Insert an indwelling catheter to accurately monitor urine output. Ordered needed for this.

Monitor potassium levels as hyperkalemia/hypokalemia will lead to an increased cardiac risk.

Adams-Stokes Syndrome

Where in the body is the complication located?

This is a heart condition.

What will the client experience?

Sudden attacks of syncope & fainting. Seizures may also be present.

What will the nurse see on the EKG/ECG?

Asystole or ventricular arrhythmias.

Is there adequate tissue perfusion during the attacks?

There will be no tissue perfusion during the attacks.

What is the treatment?

The client will need an internal pacemaker inserted during surgery.

What oral medications can be given after surgery?

Digoxin

Clinical Priorities

1. This patient is a falls risk as they will temporarily lose consciousness due to the heart skipping beats. Remember to expect fainting.

2. Epinephrine is the medication used to treat the ventricular standstill.

3. The cause of fainting is due to the lack of oxygen to the brain.

Addison's Disease

What is the cause?

A low production of hormones by the adrenal gland (glucocorticoids & mineralocorticoids).

What are some of the major symptoms?

Lethargy, weakness, and weight loss.

What color is the skin of a client with Addison's disease?

Bronzed color (hyperpigmentation) assess the palms, in the creases of skin and over pressure points.

Will this client be overweight?

No as weight loss is common.

Will the serum blood glucose levels be high or low?	Low, along with the sodium levels. Salt should be increased.
Will the serum potassium levels be high or low?	High
What is the treatment?	Lifelong glucocorticoid therapy.

Clinical Priorities

1. The three classes of adrenal corticosteroids are glucocorticoids, mineral corticoids & androgens. *All 3 classes are usually decreased.

2. An Addisonian crisis is a life-threatening emergency caused by a sudden sharp decrease in the corticosteroids. Treatment is directed toward shock management & high doses of hydrocortisone replacement. IV fluids are also administered.

3. The most common hormone therapy is *hydrocortisone* because it has glucocorticoid and mineralocorticoid properties. ☺

Allergies

Clients allergic to latex may also be allergic to which foods?	Bananas, kiwi, chestnuts.
What standard hospital equipment contains latex?	Blood pressure cuffs, gloves, stethoscopes, tourniquets, BAND-AIDs, and indwelling catheters.
Patients in which careers are most likely to develop a latex allergy?	Healthcare workers, hairdressers and mechanics
What allergy is contraindicated for IV contrast dye?	Iodine/shellfish allergy

Clinical Priorities

1. Always assess patients for allergies before giving medications.

2. If a patient is not sure if they are allergic to a medication the nurse should still administer the medication and wait 15 minutes with the patient.

3. Epinephrine is the best medication to treat anaphylactic shock on NCLEX.

Amputation

What are the major complications of having an amputation performed?	Infections, skin breakdown, phantom limb pain, and joint contractures.
What is the positioning for post-op care?	Elevate first 24 hours, then prone place client in the
-AKA (above the knee) amputation	position twice daily to prevent hip flexion.
-BKA (below the knee) amputation	Elevate foot of bed first 24 hours, then prone position twice daily to prevent hip flexion.

What should you encourage?	The expression of feelings about the lost limb.
What is phantom limb pain?	Pain felt in an area that has been amputated.

Clinical Priorities	1. A trapeze can aid in strengthening the upper extremities and allow the patient to move in bed.
	2. Initial pressure dressings and drains are removed by surgeon 48 to 72 hours postoperatively.

Anemias

Type of Anemia	Signs	Treatment
Aplastic Anemia	Decreased erythrocytes Bleeding mucous membranes Thrombocytopenia	Antilymphocyte globulin (ALG) Blood transfusions Bone marrow transplantations
Iron Deficiency Anemia	Low hemoglobin & hematocrit Pallor, fatigue, Tissue hypoxia Tachycardia *This is the most common & expected during pregnancy.	Iron supplements Dietary changes
Vitamin B 12 (Pernicious Anemia)	Pallor, "beefy red tongue" fatigue, paresthesia	Cyanocobalamin is a manufactured version of vitamin B12. Cyanocobalamin injections are needed to help the body make red blood cells. Dietary changes
Sickle Cell Anemia	See Table of Contents	You. Can. Will. Must Pass NCLEX!

Clinical Priorities	1. Diagnostics to assess for anemia: complete blood count, peripheral blood smear, bone marrow biopsy.
	2. Blood transfusions are indicated for clients who are actively bleeding or have a hemoglobin at 7 or less.
	3. Replacement iron can be administered PO or IV depending on client's condition.

Aneurysm

True or false? An aneurysm is a dilation formed at a weak point on the wall of an artery.	True
What are the symptoms of aneurysms inside the body?	Most aneurysms inside the body do not have symptoms.
What sound would be heard on auscultation?	A blowing bruit is heard.
What are some of the risk factors?	Arteriosclerosis, infection (tertiary stage of syphilis), hypertension, smoking
What is the treatment for an aneurysm?	Surgery is an option. Strict blood pressure control with medications.
What are the signs of a ruptured aneurysm?	Severe pain, N/V, tachycardia, decreased LOC, hypotension.

List important NCLEX teaching points.

Avoid straining, lifting, or exerting, take medications on schedule, report severe back and flank pain.

Clinical Priorities	1. Clients are usually asymptomatic unless the aneurysm ruptures.
	2. Non-surgical treatment focuses on maintaining blood pressure within normal limits.
	3. Surgical treatment includes a stent placement.
	4. False aneurysms can occur as a result of a vessel injury or trauma to all three layers of the artery wall.

Anorexia Nervosa

The primary symptom of illness is?

Starvation

What is the mental perception of the body?

Distorted

At what age does this disease occur?

Adolescent or teenage years

What is the usual personality type?

A perfectionist or overachiever with low esteem.

What is a major cardiac complication of anorexia?

Cardiac arrhythmias

What is a major gynecological complication of anorexia?

Amenorrhea

What is the treatment of anorexia nervosa?

Small, frequent meals with counseling and milieu therapy

Clinical Priorities	1. Anorexia is a behavioral issue to therapy must address the behavior.
	2. Two factors of treatment- nutritional rehabilitation & psychotherapy.
	3. Clients with anorexia are at risk for refeeding syndrome. This is a clinical complication that can occur due to fluid and electrolyte shifts during nutritional rehabilitation of the malnourished client.
	4. Anorexic clients with distorted thoughts about their body image do not respond well to pharmacotherapy. However, it responds well to cognitive behavioral therapy.
	5. This condition is sometimes confused with bulimia nervosa.

Appendicitis

Which age range is most affected with the condition?

10 - 30 years old

What is the most common sign of appendicitis?

Acute right lower abdominal pain

What are other signs and symptoms?

Loss of appetite, nausea, vomiting, low-grade temperature

The localized tenderness is found where?

McBurney's point

What are the tests to determine appendicitis?

Complete history and physical exam with WBC count -the results will be elevated.

What is the treatment for appendicitis?

Immediate surgery to remove appendix, IV antibiotics, Semi-Fowler's position. A NPO diet to rest the stomach.

What are the general treatments for any acute abdominal pain?

NPO status, no heat on the abdomen, assess abdominal distention, IV fluid therapy to prevent hydration.

Clinical Priorities

1. Another common sign for appendicitis is Rovsing's sign. This is characterized by right lower abdominal pain upon palpation of the left side of the lower abdomen.

2. Heat should not be placed on the abdomen as this could lead to the rupture of the appendix.

3. The most common imaging test that can confirm the diagnosis of appendicitis is an abdominal ultrasound.

Arterial Blood Gas

Where are most samples drawn from?

The radial artery in the wrist

How long should pressure be applied to the site after collecting a sample?

5 minutes

Which test should be performed before collecting an ABG on a client?

Allen's Test

What is a quick non-invasive substitute?

Pulse oximetry reading will tell a quick measurement of oxygenation status.

Asperger's Syndrome

This syndrome is a form of _____?

Autism

What is autism?

A developmental disorder that impairs the ability to communicate and interact.

What is the treatment for autism?

Speech therapy, physical and occupational therapy. Currently there is no medication that can cure the condition.

What does treatment improve?

Communication and the client's social skills.

Clinical Priorities

1. The first step in diagnosis is early detection.
2. The nurse should use clear statements that begin with the client's name to improve information processing.
3. Nursing care interventions should include dimming the lights and using a weighted blanket or vest.
4. Repetitive movement should be allowed.

Asthma

An obstructive airway disease caused by
_____ and _____ of the bronchioles?

Spasms, inflammation

What are the signs of asthma?

Shortness of breath, expiratory
wheezes, and possibly a cough.

When will the client experience the cough?

At night

What is the primary treatment goal?

To identify the allergen

Which medications work best for treatment?

Anti-inflammatory,
Corticosteroids bronchodilators
leukotriene modifiers and
Metered dose inhalers

Which should a nurse give first—the steroid or
Bronchodilators when treating asthma?

Bronchodilator-opens airway

What are leukotriene modifiers?

They are drugs used to block the
chemical leukotriene, which
reduces inflammation.

Clinical Priorities	1. The nurse should teach the client to practice controlling the environment. This includes avoiding asthma triggers, inflammatory factors, irritants, and pollutants.

STEPS TO USE A METERED DOSE INHALER
NCLEX Teaching Question

1. Remove the cap.
2. Shake the inhaler well before use.
3. Breathe out, away from the inhaler.
4. Bring the inhaler to the mouth. Place it in mouth between the teeth and close mouth around it.
5. Start to breathe in **slowly**. Press the top of the inhaler once and keep breathing in slowly until one has taken a full breath (three to five seconds).
6. Remove the inhaler from the mouth and hold the breath for about 10 seconds, then breathe out.

*If patients cannot tolerate a bitter taste or are experiencing side effects, they may need a spacer.
*Patients should rinse mouth after each dose to prevent thrush.   *Client should wait only one minute between each puff.

Autonomic Dysreflexia

Autonomic dysreflexia occurs in clients
with what type of an injury?

A spinal cord injury
(T-6 or above)

What can cause autonomic dysreflexia?

Stimuli such as a full bladder
or fecal impaction

Why is autonomic dysreflexia so serious?

It is life threatening due to
clients becoming extremely
HYPERTENSIVE.

What is the most common cause of it?

Urinary obstruction

What are the signs of autonomic dysreflexia?

Increase in the BP 40mm Hg, headache, bradycardia, blurred vision, & sweating

What should be done during an episode?

1st Place client in high Fowler's Check for bladder distention. Loosen restrictive clothing.

What is the treatment?

Removal of the stimuli. Client needs to void or have a bowel movement as fecal impaction may be present.

Clinical Priorities

1. The nurse should check for indwelling catheters that are kinked because urinary obstruction is the most common cause of AD.

2. Other causes of autonomic dysreflexia are increase in blood pressure, bradycardia, gooseflesh, and headache.

3. Gooseflesh is the same as goosebumps, caused by chills or a change of temperature in the client.

Bell's Palsy

Bell's palsy affects which cranial nerve?

Cranial nerve #7

What does the client with Bell's palsy suffer from?

Temporary facial paralysis that affects chewing, eating, and closing of the eyes.

What is the treatment for Bell's palsy?

- Wear an eye patch at night
- Use artificial tears
- Wear glasses to protect eyes
*Steroids reduce edema & swelling

Clinical Priorities

1. There are no specific diagnostic tests for Bell's palsy.

2. The majority of patients will have all of their symptoms go away within a few weeks to months.

3. This condition is often confused with a stroke. However, a stroke will affect the arms, legs, and gait of a patient. Bell's palsy will not.

Benign Prostatic Hyperplasia (BPH)

BPH is caused by _____?

The cause is unknown, but it's an enlargement of the prostate gland.

Because the prostate blocks the urethra opening, what will clients feel and see when they urinate?

Straining to urinate, decreased urine stream, feeling like they have to go all the time, dribbling urine.

Who usually gets BPH?

Men usually over 50

What is the best way to assess for BPH?

Digital rectal exam, physician will feel a pea-sized nodule. A blood test to detect the prostate specific antigen- (PSA). A urine test.

What is the common surgical treatment for BPH?	Transurethral resection of the prostate (TURP)
How is a TURP performed?	A scope goes through the penis and removes parts of the prostate.
After the procedure, what is the client at risk for?	Bleeding; monitor for hemorrhage.
All clients will get a _____ before a TURP.	Three-way (lumen) indwelling catheter.
What are the three lumens for?	Inflating the balloon, inflow of the solution, and outflow of the urine.
What will the doctor order to be done after a TURP?	Continuous Bladder Irrigation (CBI)
What is the goal of a bladder irrigation?	To reduce & prevent blood clots in the post-op client.
Will an incision be made during the irrigation?	No, the irrigation will be done using the indwelling catheter.
What type of fluid is used to irrigate the bladder?	Isotonic sterile saline
What color should the urine be?	Light pink during the procedure that turns to clear.
During CBI what must the client be monitored for?	Bladder distention, fluid overload, *hyponatremia, and blood loss.
If bladder spasms occur, give _____ or _____.	Belladonna/opium suppositories or oxybutynin
The best position for this client post-op is?	Lying flat because sitting up puts pressure on the bladder.
List client education discharge instructions.	Drink two to three liters of fluids daily. No lifting or straining. If bright red blood clots are present, call the doctor.

Do Kegel exercises to strengthen pelvis muscles. |

 Clinical Priorities

1. Clients in the initial stages of BPH do not have erectile dysfunction or blood in the urine.

2. Finasteride is a medication prescribed for BPH because it blocks a hormone that causes the prostate to enlarge.

3. BPH is often confused with prostate cancer however the B in BPH stands for benign meaning the condition will not spread. Prostate cancer cells will spread to other parts of the body.

Blood Administration

What must be received before a blood transfusion is started?	A signed written consent
Which blood type is considered universal and can be used for all other donors?	Type O Negative
What blood type is considered the universal recipient and can receive all blood types?	Type AB Positive
What is the most common infection spread through blood transfusions?	Hepatitis B
In order to determine donor compatibility, what test must be done?	Type and crossmatch
What must be done to determine a client's baseline before starting the transfusion?	Take the vital signs
What size IV gauge must the client have?	18G with a filter needle
How many nurses confirm the unit of blood?	2
How long after blood is removed from the blood bank's refrigerator should it be started?	30 minutes
How long must a nurse stay with the client after the transfusion is started?	15 minutes
How many mLs are in one unit of packed red blood cells?	About 250 mL
What are the signs of an adverse reaction?	Restlessness, nausea, hives, SOB, fever, chills, back pain
Why is blood administered at a slow rate?	Because running blood fast can cause fluid overload in patients.
Which drug is also used to treat anemia because it increases red blood cell production?	Epoetin alfa
Clients taking Epoetin alfa should be monitored for what?	Hypertension and seizure

Clinical Priorities

1. The nurse should get a signed consent form (unless it is an emergency)

2. Check vital signs before administration.

3. Confirm the blood order and blood type match with 2 licensed nurses before administration.

4. Monitor the client for 30 minutes. (The first 15 minutes stay in the room with the client.)

5. If a transfusion reaction occurs stop the blood but continue to run the normal saline that is hung with blood.

6. Make sure to collect urine and blood cultures from the client as soon as possible.

7. Notify the physician of the event.

Blood Pressure

What is a blood pressure?	The force of blood flowing through the arteries.
What is the recommended blood pressure?	120/80 for adults 90/60 for children 70/40 for infants
What are the top and bottom values?	Systolic and diastolic pressure
Define the terms: systolic and diastolic pressure.	Systolic – Pressure while heart beats Diastolic – Pressure while heart is at rest
Which value determines if a person has HTN?	Diastolic - If the pressure of the heart is elevated at rest, then hypertension is present.
What are the risk factors for hypertension?	African Americans, obesity, anxiety, diabetes mellitus type 2, and a smoking history.
What are the physical signs of hypertension?	Blurry vision, headache, chest pain; but remember that HTN is called a silent KILLER as most people don't have symptoms.
How can the size of the blood pressure cuff affect blood pressure reading?	If it is too small, the BP will the be higher than it really is. If the cuff is too big, the BP will be lower than it actually is.
What are some other factors that alter blood pressure?	Position of the client, caffeine intake, anxiety, and activity.
What is pulse pressure?	The difference between systolic and diastolic numbers
What is the mean arterial pressure?	Diastolic pressure (+) 1/3 of pulse pressure; this value should be greater than 60.
Before a blood pressure medication is given, always check _____ and _____?	Blood pressure and pulse rate
Hold the medication if systolic BP is less than ____ or heart rate is less than _____.	100, 60

Which classes of medications are used for HTN?	Diuretics, beta blockers, calcium channel blockers, and vasodilators.
Medications that end in "pril" are _____?	Ace inhibitors
Ace inhibitors correct heart failure by _____ after load.	Decreasing - they also promote vasodilation by inhibiting the production of angiotensin.
_____ is an adverse reaction seen with the use of ACE inhibitors.	Angioedema
Signs of angioedema are?	Swelling of the lips and mouth
Clients may also have a persistent, nagging _____.	Cough
Which is more dangerous in angioedema: a cough or swelling of the lips and mouth?	Swelling of the lips and mouth may indicate laryngeal angioedema. A compromised airway is the priority.
Medications that end in "olol" are _____?	Beta blockers
Clients who take anti-hypertensive medications should be taught what method to avoid falling?	Sit in a chair or at a bedside for 30 minutes after taking medication to adjust to a lower circulating blood pressure.
Which herbal medication is used to lower BP?	Garlic
Clients taking anti-hypertensives should avoid hot showers, baths, and weather. True or false?	True. These things can cause dizziness.
What is the best diet for a hypertensive client?	Low-sodium, low-fat DASH diet.

Breast Feeding

Breast feeding moms will often feel what while feeding the baby?	Abdominal cramps
Abdominal cramps are due to the release of?	Prolactin and oxytocin
What is the best way to burp a baby?	While he/she is sitting up
What is the infection of the breast tissue called?	Mastitis
What is the treatment for mastitis?	Antibiotics such as penicillin

Do you remember how HIV attacks the body?

| What are the benefits of breastfeeding? | Passive immunity, quicker weight loss in mother after birth, increase in bonding, economically a no cost food. |

| **Clinical Priorities** | 1. The patient should be aware that colostrum can be expressed late in pregnancy.
2. Clients with inverted nipples can still breastfeed with the help of a lactation consultant.
3. Clients should wear nursing pads to absorb leaking milk.
4. Nipples should be allowed to air dry to reduce irritation to the tissue.
5. Breastfeeding should begin as soon as possible after delivery.
6. Breastfeeding can help reduce postpartum bleeding.
7. Clients with breast implants can still breastfeed though the milk supply may be lowered. |

You will never change your life until you change something you do daily.
Your daily routine is the bases of your success! ☺

Buerger's Disease (Thromboangiitis Obliterans)

This disease is the obstruction and inflammation of blood vessels mainly where?	In the hands and feet
What are the clinical symptoms?	Pale, blue, hands and feet; They may tingle or be painful. They will be cold.
Who is most at risk for this disease?	Males who smoke or chew tobacco.
What are the treatment goals?	There is no cure, only symptom control; teach clients to stop smoking, dress appropriately for the weather, and try to reduce life stressors.

| **Clinical Priorities** | 1. Thrombosis of the superficial veins may occur as blood vessels swell.
2. Smoking cessation is the mainstay of therapy. This will stop the disease in most cases.
3. Amputation is required if severe ischemia occurs. |

Bulimia Nervosa

What is the eating cycle involved?	Eating binges followed by purging of all the foods consumed.
Will you be able to see physical changes or weight loss?	The client usually remains at a normal weight.
Besides purging, what other methods are used to lose weight?	Vomiting, enemas, drugs diuretics, diets, and laxatives.

What are the medical complications associated with bulimia nervosa?	Tooth decay, electrolyte imbalances, ulcers, cardiac arrhythmias
Safety is a concern in clients with bulimia nervosa because of _____.	Suicidal thoughts
List the treatment goals.	Encouraging talking, safety and assessing suicidal potential, establishing a diet plan, supervision during mealtime, and antidepressants may be prescribed

 Clinical Priorities

1. This condition is usually accompanied with a psychiatric disorder such as depression.
2. Cognitive behavioral therapy (CBT) has been found to be the most effective treatment.
3. Medications commonly used to treat this condition are: sertraline, escitalopram, fluvoxamine.
4. This condition is sometimes confused with anorexia nervosa.

Burns

What are the two age groups most at risk for suffering a burn injury?	Children and the elderly
What are the four types of burns?	Chemical, electrical, thermal and radiation
If the face/neck has been burned, what is the nursing priority?	Assess airway obstruction

Classification of Burns

1st degree (Superficial partial thickness)	Skin pink/red, painful (e.g., sunburn)
2nd degree (Deep partial thickness)	Skin red/white, blisters, and swelling is noted.
3rd degree (Full thickness)	Skin black/brown, edema, all layers of skin burned, grafting may be needed.
What is the formula used to determine fluid replacement for the first 24 hours?	The parkland formula
What is the Parkland formula?	4ml of lactated ringer (LR) x weight (kg) x % of body that is burned.
How much of this fluid do you give in the first eight hours?	½ of total volume
How much fluid do you give for the second eight hours?	¼ of total volume
How much fluid do you give for the third eight hours?	¼ of total volume

Should the client burst a blister?	No
Which is the best route for pain medications?	IV
Which diet is appropriate for clients with burns?	High calorie, high protein
What is a common electrolyte problem in clients with burns?	Hypokalemia or hyperkalemia; Both can be seen in clients with burns.
Due to prolonged stress, clients are at risk for which type of ulcers?	Curling's ulcers
What medication should be given before dressing changes?	Pain medication

Clinical Priorities

1. Clinical symptoms of the airway damaged by burns include smoky breath, hoarseness of the voice, wheezing, crowing, stridor, and drooling.

2. Clients should also be evaluated for carbon monoxide poisoning symptoms include: headaches, dizziness, tinnitus, and elevated carboxyhemoglobin levels.

3. There are two types of grafts to know for NCLEX:
   -**Homografts** (allografts) which are from human skin obtained from a cadaver.
   -**Heterografts** (xenografts) are obtained from another species. Pig skin is a common heterograft.

Cancer

True or false? Cancer is an abnormal growth of cells.	True – Cell growth is uncontrolled
When the cancer cell travels from the original location to a new place, what is it called?	Metastasis
What acronym is used to describe the warning signs of cancer?	**C.A.U.T.I.O.N.**
What do the letters stand for?	**C**hange in bowel or bladder **A**ny sore that does not heal **U**nusual bleeding/discharge **T**hickening in breast **I**ndigestion **O**bvious change in a wart **N**agging cough or hoarseness
What are the two ways to describe a tumor?	By grading or staging
What is the difference between the two?	Grading describes a tumor by the cells. Staging describes the progression of a tumor by the clinical symptoms.
What are the three types of radiation treatment?	External unsealed; internal sealed; and internal
What precautions must be taken for a client receiving radiation treatment?	Private room and a bathroom Limit visitors, rotate nursing staff who provide care, place a sign at door and bedside

What is the most dangerous type of radiation?

Sealed internal radiation because a solid radioactive implant is placed inside of the tumor.

What additional precautions must be taken for clients receiving sealed internal radiation?

All body fluids are radioactive; use hazardous clean up gloves and gown.

If a client's sealed internal implant falls out. (e.g., cervical implant), what should you do?

Pick it up with long-handle forceps and put it in a lead container.

Chemotherapy works by destroying the cell _____.

Wall

What are the side effects of chemotherapy?

Nausea, anorexia, alopecia sterility, oral thrush, neuropathy, fatigue

Why is metoclopramide given?

To reduce nausea

Is alopecia from chemotherapy permanent?

No, it is temporary

Is sterility from chemotherapy permanent?

Yes

Clients with cancer will also need ____ _____.

Neutropenic precautions

What are neutropenic precautions?

Strict hand washing
No visitors who are sick
No children allowed
No raw food, no live plants
No free-standing water in the room.

What is filgrastim?

A drug used to treat neutropenia; the nurse should monitor WBCs after administration.

When is the best time to do a breast self-exam?

Once a month however these are no longer recommended due to the harm of false positive results

When is the best time to do a self-testicular exam?

The same day each month

If a client has had a mastectomy, can a nurse take a blood pressure on the affected side?

No they cannot have an IV or have a blood pressure taken on the affected side.

List some other post-mastectomy client education tips.

Elevate affected extremity, no initial exercise after surgery, encourage discussion for positive self-image.

Clinical Priorities	1. The staging of a tumor uses the letters TNM
	    T - <u>T</u>umor (size, location, origin)
	    N - Lymph <u>N</u>ODES (involvement of regional and distant)
	    M - <u>M</u>etastasis or spread of the disease.
	2. It is important to note that a biopsy of a tumor does not remove the tumor.
	3. *Chemotherapy* is the use of antineoplastic agents.
	4. *Immunotherapy* is the strengthening of the immune system.
	5. *Systemic therapy* is chemotherapy + immunotherapy where treatment focuses on the entire body.
	6. *Concurrent therapy* is radiation therapy + chemotherapy.
	7. *Neoadjuvant therapy* is therapy prior to a surgery.
	8. *Adjuvant therapy* is sometimes called "helper" therapy in addition to a treatment (such as surgery).
	9. The cytopenias of chemotherapy are low: white blood cells, red blood cells, platelets.

ReMar NCLEX Planner Page

Two awesome things that happened today:
1.
2.

Two struggles I have encountered while studying:
1.
2.

Possible solutions for these struggles:
1.
2.

I am proud that:

Tomorrow will be a great day because:

You've got this!
Stay focused and remember your WHY!

You Can. You Will. You Must.
PASS NCLEX!

Professor Regina M. Callion MSN, RN

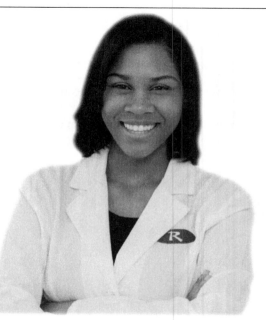

Cardiopulmonary Resuscitation (CPR)

CPR	Infant (up to 1 year)	Child (1 year to signs of puberty)	Older Child & Adult (puberty and older)
Verify Scene Safety	Do not enter an unsafe environment. Call 9-1-1		
Check the victim's responsiveness	If the victim is unresponsive, shout for help. Call 9-1-1 with a mobile device, if outside the hospital. Send someone to find an AED.		
Activate 9-1-1	If the nurse is alone and does not have access to a mobile device leave the victim to call 9-1-1 or activate EMS first, then look for an AED. Return to perform CPR.		
Determine if victim is breathing & has a pulse	Simultaneously check for breathing and pulse for no more than 10 seconds. Note: Agonal breaths are not considered signs of breathing. For children and infants, a pulse rate of less than 60 beats/minute is treated as no pulse.		
	Check brachial artery on the inside of the victim's upper arm near the armpit	Check the carotid artery on the victim's the neck. Use the side closest to you.	
Rescue breathing **If victim has a DEFINITE detectable pulse but is not breathing.**	1 breath every 3-5 seconds Check pulse again every 2 minutes. If pulse is less than 60 beats per minute, or perfusion remains poor add chest compressions.	1 breath every 5-6 seconds Check pulse every 2 minutes. *For suspected opioid overdose, administer naloxone, if available.	
If the victim has no detectable pulse. **BEGIN CPR**	1 rescuer: 30 compressions: 2 breaths 2+ rescuers: 15 compressions: 2 breaths Use AED as soon as it arrives	1 rescuer: 30 compressions: 2 breaths 2+ rescuers: 15 compressions: 2 breaths Use AED as soon as it arrives	
Compression rate	100-120 compression per minute		
Hand placement	1 rescuer: 2 fingers 2+ rescuers: 2 thumbs on the center of the chest just below the nipple line.	2 hands on the lower half of the breastbone	
Compression depth	1/3 the depth of the chest about 1.5 inches	2 to 2.4 inches	
Chest recoil	Look for full chest recoil after each compression		

Cataracts

What are the signs of cataracts?	Milky or white lens Painless blurry vision
How are cataracts treated?	No treatment required until the vision is severely impaired.
During surgery, what is done?	The cataracts are removed and a new lens may be implanted.
After surgery, will the vision be corrected?	Only if a new lens is placed. If no lens is placed, the client will still need glasses or contacts.
After surgery, what is the main concern?	To check for hemorrhage of the eye. The nurse should place the client in semi-Fowler's position
What do you tell clients to avoid after surgery?	Coughing, sneezing, bending over at the waist, straining, rubbing eye, or crying. Also no lifting weight greater than five pounds.
How should the client sleep after surgery?	They should sleep on the unaffected side. If surgery was done on both eyes, clients should sleep on the back. The client should use an eye shield at night to protect the eye.

Clinical Priorities	1. Before surgery the nurse should hold anticoagulant therapy to prevent ocular hemorrhage.
	2. Before surgery dilating eye drops may be prescribed.
	3. After surgery steroid eye drops may be prescribed.

Celiac Disease

Foods containing _____ must not be eaten.	Gluten (This is a protein.)
In Celiac's disease, malabsorption of _____ occurs.	Fats
What foods contain gluten?	B.R.O.W. (barley, rye, oats, and wheat)
The client's abdomen is often _____.	Distended
What does the client's stool look like?	Smelly, pale, bulky; expect lots of gas with some diarrhea.

The best food substitutes are _____ and _____.	Corn, rice
Can a client on a gluten free diet have cookies, spaghetti, or waffles?	No all these products have grains/gluten in them.
What is another name for celiac disease?	Celiac sprue

<table>
<tr><td rowspan="4">Clinical Priorities</td><td>1. Some non-food items may contain gluten (beauty and personal care products, children's toys (finger paint & play dough).</td></tr>
<tr><td>2. The challenges of malnutrition are: weight loss, fatigue, dental issues, failure to thrive.</td></tr>
<tr><td>3. Avoid: Overfeeding the client which can cause abdominal pain. The nurse should also avoid offering cold drinks which can make abdominal cramps and diarrhea worse.</td></tr>
<tr><td>4. Anticipated medication orders:

[] Antidiarrheals – loperamide   [] Stimulants – amphetamine
[] Antispasmodics – hyoscine   [] NSAIDs – naproxen</td></tr>
</table>

Cerebrovascular Accident (CVA)

Define the term CVA.	Reduction of cerebral blood flow and oxygen which causes brain cell damage.
The three most common causes of CVA are _____?	Embolism, hemorrhage, and thrombus
What are the signs of a CVA?	Client reports headache, nausea, nuchal rigidity, HTN, a slow bounding pulse, Cheyne-Stokes respirations, speech change, and facial droop
What is the difference between CVA and a Transient Ischemic Attack (TIA)?	TIA is a temporary period of neurological deficit with similar signs as CVA but the symptoms will all resolve and disappear.
What is agnosia?	Inability to use object correctly.
Expressive aphasia occurs when _____.	The client cannot communicate properly. The aphasia can be expressive or receptive.
If the left hemisphere of the brain is affected, you will see weakness on the____ side.	Right
If the right hemisphere is affected, you will see weakness on the____ side.	Left
Remember to place the client's belongings on the _____ side.	Unaffected

The tests used to determine a CVA are?

CT, EEG, & cerebral arteriography

Patients with hemorrhagic stroke are at an increased risk for which complication?

Seizures due to possible bleeding in the cerebral cortex.

What are the nursing assessments?

Monitor vital signs, neuro checks, watch for seizures, monitor for an increase in cranial pressure, check ability to swallow (risk for aspiration)

What complication of the eyes can a client with a CVA have?

Corneal abrasion- as the lacrimal glands will not produce lubrication.

What is the activity level for this client?

Strict bed rest

How should the room environment be?

Quiet, peaceful, with objects within reach on unaffected side

How do you position the CVA client?

Turn every two hours on the unaffected side, then 20 minutes on the affected side, make sure to elevate affected extremities.

Why would a thrombolytic be given?

To dissolve a clot

Do not give thrombolytics if the cause of the stroke is _____.

Hemorrhage-this will cause more bleeding in the client

What other medications may be prescribed to treat a CVA?

Anti-hypertensives, anti-coagulants (not for a hemorrhagic stroke) and anti-convulsant medications.

Do anti-coagulants like coumadin and aspirin dissolve blood clots?

No, they only thin the blood; they do not dissolve blood clots.

Clinical Priority	1. A CT scan is the initial diagnostic test performed to determine the type of stroke the client has.
	2. Pupil reactions are regulated by the cranial nerve 3 oculomotor. This evaluates an intact brain stem
	3. Nuchal rigidity may indicate meningeal irritation. Seizures may reflect an increase in ICP.
	4. When turning the patient, the head should be slightly elevated to reduce arterial pressure and promote venous drainage.
	5. Cluster nursing care and restrict visitors because continuous stimulation or activity can increase intracranial pressure.
	6. Anticipated medication orders:
	Thrombolytics: tissue plasminogen activator (tPA)
	Anticoagulants: warfarin sodium, low molecular weight heparin
	Antiplatelets: aspirin, ticlopidine
	Antifibrinolytics: aminocaproic acid

Chronic Obstructive Pulmonary Disorder (COPD)

What are the three disorders that make up COPD?

Asthma, bronchitis, & emphysema

What are the clinical signs of COPD?

Shortness of breath (SOB), activity wheezing, a productive cough and cyanosis.

What would the arterial blood gas show?

Hypoxemia

What does the chest of a client with COPD look like?

Barrel chest

What would the fingers of a COPD client look like?

Clubbed fingers

Due to SOB with activity clients may experience _____ because of difficulty eating.

Weight loss

Why must you assess the amount of O2 your COPD client receives?

The client keep high levels of carbon dioxide in their blood stream which controls the rate of their breathing.

A client with COPD should not receive O2 by NC greater than _____.

2 LPM

To control SOB, the ___ ___ ___ technique should be taught.

Pursed lip breathing

Clinical Priorities

1. COPD is often confused with congestive heart failure, bronchiectasis, or tuberculosis.

2. Smoking is the primary cause of this condition. The client should be educated on the benefits of completely stopping tobacco.

3. The nurse should avoid chest physiotherapy in COPD exacerbation which can cause bronchoconstriction.

4. Anticipated medication orders:

   Bronchodilator: inhaled ipratropium bromide

   Corticosteroid: prednisone

   Beta 2 agonists: albuterol

Chronic Renal Failure

Chronic renal failure is progressive and irreversible. True or false?

True

What are possible causes of CRF?

Hypertension, frequent infections, diabetes mellitus type 2 and renal obstruction

What clinical signs would clients show?

Decreased urine, hypertension, decreased urine specific gravity, and fluid overload.

What is uremic frost?	Urea crystals that come through the skin with perspiration
Where would you see this frost?	Face, underarms, groin; teach the client to wash their skin with plain water.
What are the nursing interventions for chronic renal failure?	Modification of diet, diuretics anti-hypertensives, monitor BUN & creatinine, and taking a daily weight. The weight should be taken at the same time each day.
Clients may need _____ to assist with waste removal in the blood.	Dialysis
What is the best diet for CRF patients?	Moderate carbohydrate, low protein; the goal of this diet is to provide energy while decreasing protein metabolism.

Clinical Priorities
1. Monitor clients for anemia, as erythropoietin production decreases in end stage renal disease.
2. Monitor fluid intake, fluid restriction may be necessary.
3. Monitor the patient's access site for patency. See dialysis section for further instruction.

Corticosteroids

Most corticosteroids end in _____.	- ONE
What are the primary functions of corticosteroids?	To decrease inflammation and hormone replacement
What should you teach clients about stopping corticosteroid therapy?	To gradually decrease use; don't abruptly stop
What must be monitored while a client is taking a steroid?	Potassium levels which will decrease. Glucose levels which will increase. Sodium levels will increase as well as overall fluid retention. This may cause an increase in blood pressure.
Corticosteroids may cause symptoms of _____.	Cushing's syndrome.
Corticosteroids will also delay _____ healing.	Wound
If the client is NPO before surgery should the nurse still give the steroid?	Yes, request the doctor to change the route because surgery can cause additional stress on the body and steroids will help in the recovery process.

Corticosteroids

Short Acting Drugs		
Medication	Administration	Duration
Hydrocortisone	Oral, parenteral, topical	8-12 hours
Cortisone	Oral parenteral, topical	8-12 hours

Intermediate Acting Drugs		
Medication	Administration	Duration
Methyl-prednisolone	Oral, parenteral, topical	12-36 hours
Prednisolone*	Eye drops, Oral parenteral, topical	12-36 hours
Prednisone*	Oral prep only	12-36 hours

Long-Acting Drugs		
Medication	Administration	Duration
Bethamethasone	Oral, parenteral	24-72 hours
Dexamethasone	Eye drops, parenteral	24-72 hours

Clinical Priorities

1. Teach the client the signs of corticosteroid deficiency and excess.
2. Oral use of this medication may cause oral candidiasis (thrush).
3. Oral use may also cause irritation to the lining of upper gastrointestinal tract.
4. Medication should be taken with food or milk.
5. Clients should monitor their salt intake.
6. This medication should not be abruptly discontinued but clients should taper off the medication.

COVID-19

Is this a viral or bacterial condition?

It is a viral condition

What is the virus called?

Severe acute respiratory syndrome coronavirus 2 (SARS-CoV-2)

How soon do symptoms appear?

Symptoms appear 2-14 days after exposure to the virus.

Which isolation precaution is required?

The mode of transmission is human to human via respiratory droplets. So droplet precaution is required.

What are the signs of a COVID-19 infection?

Nasal congestion, sneezing, respiratory distress, cough, headache. Diarrhea, smell or taste changes may occur. The spectrum of symptoms range from asymptomatic to respiratory failure.

How is COVID-19 diagnosed?

There are 2 types of viral tests used to make the diagnosis of COVID-19.

What are the tests?

1. Nucleic acid amplification Test (NAATs)
2. Antigen tests

What is the treatment for COVID-19?

Nirmatrelvir – ritonavir is a combination drug that should be administered within five days of symptom onset.

Clinical Priorities	1. Viral particles are released when an infected person coughs, sneezes, or talks.
	2. Infection might also occur if a person's hands are contaminated by these secretions and another person touches a shared surface.
	3. COVID-19 is a hypercoagulable state associated with an increased risk for venous thromboembolism. This includes deep vein thrombosis and pulmonary embolism.
	4. "Long-COVID" is referred to as post-COVID conditions that develop during or after an acute COVID-19 illness that continue for greater than 2 months.
	5. Nirmatrelvir – ritoavir should not be administered to clients with severe kidney impairment.

Cranial Nerves

What nerve	What it controls
I Olfactory	Sense of smell
II Optic	Vision
III Oculomotor IV Trochlear VI Abducens	Eye movement
V Trigeminal	Sensations of the face
VII Facial	Expressions of the face
VIII Acoustic	Hearing and balance
IX Glossopharyngeal	Gag and swallow
X Vagus	Gag and parasympathetic
XI Spinal Accessory	Back and neck muscles
XII Hypoglossal	Tongue

The client is unable to shrug his shoulders; which nerve is dysfunctional?

CN X1 Accessory

A client is unable to smell his morning coffee; which nerve is dysfunctional?

CN 1 Olfactory

A client is unable to distinguish between salty and sweet tastes; which nerve is dysfunctional?

CN VII Facial

Which is responsible for the control of the heart rate and digestive system?

CN X Vagus

Crohn's Disease

Crohn's disease is an _____ of the bowels.

Inflammation

Can Crohn's disease be cured with surgery?

No, symptoms frequently will reoccur.

Crohn's disease affects the digestive tract from the mouth to anus. True or false?

True

What are the symptoms of Crohn's disease?

Abdominal pain, diarrhea, weight loss

Excessive diarrhea will cause which electrolyte imbalance?

Hypokalemia

What foods should be avoided and why?

Dairy products and high-fiber meals, which may worsen diarrhea.

Crohn's disease can lead to which kind of cancer?

Colon

What are the treatment goals?

Drugs and nutrition to reduce inflammation.

Clinical Priorities

1. The client has a high risk for malnutrition, malabsorption, and dehydration.

2. Expect intermittent bouts of low-grade fever, diarrhea, and right lower quadrant pain.

3. Anticipated orders:

    Supplemental enteral therapy by nasogastric tube.

    TPN is utilized only if high-grade blockage of the intestines or fistulas are present.

    Anti-inflammation: aminosalicylates

Cushing's Syndrome

What is the cause?

A high production of hormones by the adrenal glands. (Glucocorticoids)

What are some major symptoms?

Buffalo hump, moon face, hirsutism lethargy, weakness, and weight gain

What is the skin of a client with Cushing's syndrome like?

Fragile & bruises easily.

Will this client be overweight?

Yes weight gain is common.

Will the serum blood glucose levels be high or low?

High, the sodium levels will also be increased.

Will the serum potassium levels be high or low?

Low as will the calcium levels be decreased too.

What is the treatment?

Possible hypophysectomy or adrenalectomy then lifelong glucocorticoid therapy.

<table>
<tr><td rowspan="1">Clinical Priorities</td><td>

1. Anticipated laboratory values:

Dexamethasone suppression test-The client will be given dexamethasone which should lower the blood cortisol levels however in Cushing's the levels will remain high.

Late night salivary cortisol test-Late at night the cortisol levels in the saliva should be the lowest however in Cushing's the levels will remain high. The samples are taken at midnight.

2. The client has a high risk for fluid overload. This may lead to pulmonary edema and heart failure.

3. The nurse should monitor bone density as the client is at risk for osteoporosis.

4. The prevention of opportunistic infections should be a part of the care plan as the client has a low functioning immune system.
</td></tr>
</table>

Cystic Fibrosis

In cystic fibrosis, the _____ or exocrine glands are affected.

mucus producing glands

How does cystic fibrosis abnormally change mucus gland secretions?

The mucus will become sticky and cause obstructions.

What are the two systems most affected by cystic fibrosis?

Respiratory-the mucus gets trapped in the lungs.

Digestive- the mucus blocks the pancreas and digestive enzymes, making the absorption of nutrients very difficult.

What is the most accurate test for cystic fibrosis?

Sweat test - the chloride level will be greater than 60 mEq/L.

What are other ways to diagnose cystic fibrosis?

Chest x-ray, stool analysis, and a pulmonary function test.

How does poor absorption of fat in the digestive tract change the appearance of stool?

It causes steatorrhea (greasy, foul-smelling, pale stool)

_____ are given with each meal to help with the absorption of nutrients.

Pancreatic enzymes

What is the most appropriate diet for cystic fibrosis?

High calorie, high protein

_____ is a common technique used to clear thick mucus from the lungs. This is important for preventing respiratory infections.

Postural drainage

What should parents who already have a child with cystic fibrosis do before having another child?

They should get genetic counseling because cystic fibrosis is hereditary.

> **Clinical Priorities**
> 1. Clients with cystic fibrosis lose excessive amounts of salt when they sweat which can cause abnormal heart rhythms.
> 2. The "6 foot" rule should be followed where clients remain a 6-foot distance between people who are sick and other clients with cystic fibrosis.
> 3. Two cystic fibrosis clients should not be placed in the same room as the spreading of new germs may cause aggressive lung infections.
> 4. Immunizations and yearly flu and COVID-19 shots are recommended.

Diabetic Teaching

Which type of diabetes is controlled mostly by diet and exercise?

Diabetes mellitus type 2

Which type of diabetes is controlled mostly by insulin?

Diabetes mellitus type 1

What should the nurse teach diabetic Patients about foot care?

Have the doctor cut the toe nails straight across. Inspect the feet daily for sores. Keep the skin clean and dry.

If a diabetic vomits after taking PO anti-diabetic medication what should they do?

Monitor blood sugar and do not repeat dose. The medication may have been absorbed.

How often should a diabetic get an eye exam?

Yearly as diabetes can cause retinopathy.

What is insulin lipodystrophy?

It is the result of not rotating SQ insulin injection sites. If the client injects in the same place repeatedly, a fatty mass will appear, decreasing insulin absorption in that area. Teach injection site rotation.

Should the patient aspirate if injecting insulin SQ?

No

What is the primary injection site for insulin?

Abdomen

Exercising _____ blood glucose levels.

Lowers

Alcohol, oral contraceptives, aspirin, and MAOIs _____ blood glucose.

Lower

Infection, dehydration, stress, and surgery _____ blood glucose levels.

Increase

What should the nurse give to the client who is hypoglycemic and UNCONSCIOUS?	Glucagon (IV or IM)
Insulin pumps that are wearable mimic which organ?	Pancreas
What is the insulin used in the wearable insulin pump?	Regular or short-acting
How often is the insertion site changed when a patient wears an insulin pump?	Every 2 to 3 days
Is the insulin delivered continuous or intermittently?	Continuous
What should clients be advised not to do while wearing an insulin pump?	Smoke cigarettes or drink alcohol

Clinical Priorities (See this subject also in the V2 lectures under Diabetes Overview for more information)	1. Inform the client to monitor glycosylated hemoglobin or HbA1C. This is a blood test that shows the average blood sugar level for 3 months time.
	2. The client's knowledge should be assessed related to diabetes care. This includes limiting carbohydrate intake, exercise, and medications because of these affect blood glucose levels.
	3. Clients should be advised that an intake of only "sugar-free" foods will not control blood glucose levels as carbohydrates influence blood glucose levels.
	4. Complications of diabetes mellitus is neuropathy, retinopathy, and nephropathy.

Dialysis

What are the 2 types of dialysis?	1. Hemodialysis 2. Peritoneal dialysis (PD)
What is the purpose of hemodialysis?	It removes nitrogenous waste products, excess fluid and electrolytes from the blood by means of an artificial kidney.
What are the two types of hemodialysis accesses available to clients?	Grafts and shunts

Hemodialysis Access	Grafts	Shunts	Central Venous Catheter
What is the purpose?	To connect the patient's bloodstream to the dialysis machine.	To connect the patient's bloodstream to the dialysis machine.	An emergency access site for immediate dialysis
What is it?	A synthetic tube that is surgically placed under the skin, connecting an *artery* to a *vein*. Will be written as "AV graft"	Also known as a *fistula*, a surgical connection of an *artery* and a *vein* in the arm creating a natural access site. *It is made of the patient's own tissue. Will be written as "AV fistula"	A flexible long tube that is threaded through the skin into a central vein in the neck, chest, or groin.
How soon can it be used for dialysis?	3-6 weeks	1 to 4 months	Immediate use
How long does it last?	Approximately 2-3 years	Gold Standard 10 years or more	Should be removed quickly. May damage central veins.
Nursing interventions	This is best if a client has blocked or damaged veins. Requires needles to access the graft. Fistulas are more likely to be useable when they meet the rule of 6's -Flow greater than -600 mL/min -Diameter at least 0.6 -No more than 0.6 cm deep. Nurses and patients should wear a surgical mask during connect and disconnect procedures. Nurses should wear gloves.	Listen for the sound of blood flowing through the AV fistula. This is called a "bruit" and indicates the AV fistula is working. Also, a vibration can be felt on the overlying skin, this is referred to as a "thrill." This is also an indication of proper function. This access may require another type of temporary access during the healing and maturation phase. Needles are required to access the AV fistula for hemodialysis. Nurses and patients should wear a surgical mask during connect and disconnect procedures. Nurses should wear gloves.	Teach the client this type of access can increase the length of hemodialysis treatment. Heparin is used to maintain permeability. Complications of frequent heparin administration are alopecia, allergic reactions, thrombocytopenia, and bleeding. Nurses and patients should wear a surgical mask during connect and disconnect procedures. Nurses should wear gloves.

Which one lasts longer a graft or shunt?   AV shunts/fistulas

Which one is prone to blood clots
a graft or a shunt?   AV grafts

Which one is MORE prone to infection
a graft or a shunt?   A graft requires more
                                                            frequent monitoring.

What are the clinical signs of infection
of the hemodialysis access?   Redness, swelling, and
                                                            drainage.

How long does hemodialysis take to complete?   3-5 hours

What is the purpose of peritoneal dialysis?   It removes nitrogenous waste
                                                            products, excess fluid and
                                                            electrolytes from the blood by
                                                            means of the peritoneal membrane.

Peritoneal dialysis access	PD catheter
What is the purpose?	A catheter which uses the lining of the abdomen (peritoneum) and a dialysate solution to clean the blood.
What is it?	A flexible hollow tube about the size of a straw that is surgically placed in the abdomen.
How soon can it be used for dialysis?	Although it can be used immediately it is best to wait 10-14 days for the catheter site to heal.
How long does it last?	Many years
Nursing interventions?	Teach clients to practice good hand hygiene. Clients should avoid clothing that is too tight. Access sites should be inspected daily for signs of infection. Teach the client that the solution will have to stay in the abdomen for 4 to 6 hours. This is called the "dwell time."

What are the advantages of PD?

Dialysis can be performed at home. It takes less time to finish. Clients should wear a mask when accessing port site.

Does blood leave the body with PD?

No, the patient's blood does not leave the body.

During the client's dwell time can they move around?

Yes, the client is free to move around and go about their normal activities.

How long does dwell time last?

It can be 4-6 hours. The exchange of solution is 30-40 minutes.

What is the name of the infection that can develop in the abdomen as a result of PD?

Peritonitis

What are the clinical signs of peritonitis?

1. A swollen/distended abdomen
2. Pain and tenderness in abdomen
3. Dialysis drain fluid that is cloudy
4. An exit site that is red and has pus
5. Fever, nausea, and vomiting

How is peritonitis treated?

Antibiotics, it is possible for the antibiotics to be put inside of the dialysate solution

Domestic Violence

What are signs of domestic violence in children?

Frequent bruises or burns, shrinking back when an adult approaches and hitting others.

What two factors play an important part in domestic violence?

Power and control, as the abuser sees the victim as a a possession.

What are the various types of abuse?

Physical, verbal, emotional, sexual and financial

What are signs of neglect in children?

Stealing food, lack of dental care, poor hygiene, poor school attendance, saying that no one is home.

When a victim of rape shows no emotion or feelings after an attack, what is this called?	Controlled pattern response
What are the 5 stages of domestic violence in an intimate relationship?	Honeymoon stage, build-up of stress, anger, beating, and then reconciliation.
Should a rape victim take a shower before coming to the hospital for treatment?	No physical evidence may be washed away in the shower.
If a client comes into the hospital afraid for their life due to domestic abuse, should the nurse suggest they do not return home?	Yes the nurse should help the client explore other housing options.
What is sexual abuse by a family member called?	Incest

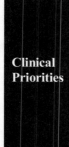

Clinical Priorities

1. Nurses are mandated reporters and must report any abuse of minors, elders, or vulnerable groups.

2. If the victim is with the suspected abuser the nurse should separate the victim from the abuser during the examination.

3. The nurse should report suspicion of abuse to the doctor or healthcare provider first.

4. Domestic violence screening questions include:
"Do you feel safe at home?"
"Does your partner ever make you feel afraid?"
"Have you ever been hit, slapped, kicked, or otherwise physically hurt by your partner?"

Donning Sterile Gloves

Gather all of the necessary supplies.
Wash and dry hands.
Place package on a dry waist-high surface.
Open package using outer one-inch margin, facing gloves toward you.
With two fingers on the non-dominant hand, pick up cuff of first glove.
Place glove on dominant hand.
Slide gloved fingers into the cuff of the other sterile glove.
Place the non-dominant hand into the glove, making sure not to touch the outside of the glove.
With both hands gloved, touch only the sterile area to adjust the gloves for comfort.

Epiglottitis

What is the epiglottis and what does it do?	A flap of skin at the base of tongue. It opens & closes during breathing.
What is the cause of epiglottitis?	Haemophilus influenza
Is this caused by a virus or bacteria?	Bacteria
What is the usual age of children who get epiglottitis?	2 - 5 years old
What are the signs of epiglottitis?	4 D's (Drooling, Dysphagia, Dysphonia [no voice] and Distress)
What will the child look like during an episode of epiglottitis?	Sitting upright; drooling, shallow, rapid breathing, a protruding tongue is seen.

Can epiglottitis be treated at home?	No, the child must go to the hospital immediately.
When assessing the airway should a tongue depressor or tongue blade be used?	NO, NEVER put anything in the mouth to assess!
If the child cannot breathe, what might be done?	Intubation
Which medication will be given to treat epiglottitis?	Antibiotic therapy
How can epiglottitis be avoided?	By getting the H. influenza vaccine

Clinical Priorities

1. In acute epiglottitis the "thumb sign" is indicative of an irrevocable loss of airway. The normal epiglottis is a thin, curved flap of soft tissue however during epiglottitis, it becomes swollen and enlarged to appear as big as a thumb.

2. Other clinical signs to be expected are high fever, sore throat, and a muffled voice. The muffled voice can also be called a "Hot Potato Voice."

3. This condition is sometimes confused with croup. Croup does cause airway obstruction, but it has a slow onset whereas epiglottitis is a rapid progression to airway obstruction.

Genital Herpes

How is genital herpes spread?	During sexual contact or birth
What are the symptoms for males?	Painful, vesicular lesions
What are the symptoms for females?	Painful, vesicular lesions
Are these lesions always present on the body?	No, they come and go.
If lesions are present in a pregnant woman, how should she deliver?	C-section
What triggers outbreaks of genital herpes?	Stress, anxiety, sunlight fatigue, and illness
How often should a woman with herpes get a pap smear?	Every six months
Can genital herpes be cured? What is the treatment?	No cure. Acyclovir

Clinical Priorities

1. Abstinence is the only guaranteed protection against genital herpes.

2. Neonatal herpes is a potentially deadly infection because the immune system of the infant is not fully developed. The herpes virus can cause brain and spinal cord damage. The virus can also attack the liver, lungs, and kidneys.

3. Acyclovir can be prescribed the last month of pregnancy to prevent active lesions during the time of delivery.

Gestational Diabetes

What causes it?

Gestational diabetes is caused by hormonal changes during pregnancy that affect insulin sensitivity.

What are the risk factors?

Maternal age over 25
Patients who are obese
Patients who have been pregnant multiple times

At what point in pregnancy does it begin?

Second to third trimester

Does it go away after delivery?

Yes, the condition should resolve and blood glucose levels return to normal.

What are the clinical symptoms?

Increased hunger and thirst
Frequent urination
Recurrent infections
Dry mouth itchy skin
However often the patient cannot distinguish the signs, which is why every pregnant woman is screened.

Is exercise recommended during pregnancy?

Regular physical activity is important in maintaining a healthy blood glucose level during pregnancy.

How is gestational diabetes treated?

Mother: Daily blood sugar monitoring, healthy diet, and exercise.
Fetus: a non-stress test may be ordered.

Which antidiabetic medication is safe to give?

Insulin is the first line choice. Metformin is also safe to administer.
Glyburide is also safe to administer.

What is macrosomia?

It is the term for a newborn with a larger than average weight.

What are the nursing considerations for macrosomia?

This infant has an increased for injuries during birth. For example shoulder dystocia, bone fractures and brachial plexus injury.

The infant with macrosomia is at a high risk for?

- Hypoglycemia
- Jaundice
- Respiratory distress
*These babies are big but they require extra health monitoring.

What are the clinical signs of newborn hypoglycemia?

Jitteriness, apnea, cyanosis and tachypnea.

What is the treatment for newborn hypoglycemia?

Oral milk feedings are the initial intervention. Buccal dextrose gel can also be given when the symptoms are mild. In severe cases IV dextrose is administered.

Clinical Priorities

1. Infants with an increased size should have frequent blood glucose monitoring due to risk for hypoglycemia.

2. A heel stick is used to obtain the blood sample from a newborn.

3. Surfactant and supplemental oxygen are administered for infants with respiratory distress. Glucose levels in newborn require treatment when the number is less than 50 mg/dL during the first 24 hours of life. Or after 2 days old when the glucose level is less than 60 mg/dL. Any infant that is symptomatic should also be treated for hypoglycemia.

4. Testing for gestational diabetes is usually done between 24-28 weeks in pregnancy.

Glaucoma

How does glaucoma affect vision?

It becomes blurry and the patient experiences tunnel vision. There will also be halos around the light.

This condition can be acute or chronic due to _____.

Increased intraocular pressure

_____ is the simple, painless procedure used to measure intraocular pressure.

Tonometry

What are the two types of glaucoma?

Open angle and closed angled

Which one is painful?

Closed angle is painful but it is not the most common of the two.

State the class of drug used to constrict the pupil and let aqueous hum.

Miotics

Give an example of a miotic medication?

Timolol or pilocarpine

Why might diuretics be given to clients with glaucoma?

To decrease aqueous humor production.

Which diuretic is usually prescribed?

Osmitrol because it dehydrates or draws water out of the vitreous humor.

Never give _____ because they dilate the pupils.

Mydriatics

If surgery is required, what should be monitored for post-operatively?

Hemorrhage

What post-op teaching should be done?

No straining, heavy lifting, crying, or rubbing the eyes.

Clinical Priorities

1. The goal of therapy is to prevent further deterioration of the vision. This is done by lowering intraocular pressure.

2. The client must be educated on how to properly administer eye drops. The focus should be put on counting the correct amount of drops and adhering to the schedule.

3. The nurse should assist with medication education:
   Direct-acting topical miotic drops cause pupillary constriction.
   Beta blockers decrease the formation of aqueous humor without changing the pupil size or vision. Remember beta blockers are contraindicated if patients have bradycardia or asthma.
   *Acetazolamide belongs to the carbonic anhydrase inhibitors and also decreases the production of fluid inside of the eye.

4. Patients should get an ophthalmic (eye) assessment every three months.

Hyperbilirubinemia

What is considered an elevated serum bilirubin level?

> Serum levels higher than 12mg/dl.

What are the clinical signs of this condition?

> The condition presents with excess bilirubin in the bloodstream. Dark colored urine. Pale clay colored stool can also be present if the liver is the source of the issue.

What will a newborn's skin look like?

> Jaundice –a yellow pigment usually seen on first day of life. Adults will also present with yellowing of the skin and sclera.

Why does the skin and sclera turn yellow?

> Because bilirubin is yellow.

What is bilirubin?

> Bilirubin is the yellow substance that the body creates when red blood cells are broken down.

What is the treatment for increased bilirubin levels?

> Phototherapy for newborns. Breastfeeding or increased feedings should also be encouraged. Adult jaundice usually isn't treated.

> The focus is on the condition causing the jaundice. Once that condition is treated the jaundice goes away.

Clinical Priorities

1. Jaundice in newborns is normal. At birth the newborn's liver is not fully developed to remove all the bilirubin. However, jaundice in adults is always caused by a disease process.

2. Phototherapy is a commonly used treatment for neonatal jaundice. Phototherapy is exposing the baby's skin to light. The light helps break down the excess bilirubin into a form that can be excreted from the body more easily.

3. Babies undergoing phototherapy require frequent monitoring of their temperature and hydration.

4. The baby should be 18 inches away from the light while wearing a diaper only. Prolonged exposure to blue light can cause retinal damage. The eyes of the newborn should be covered.

Huntington's Disease

What kind of disease is this?

It is an inherited disorder in which the nerve cells in the brain breakdown.

Which organ is most affected?

The brain because neurons die which control various body movements.

What are symptoms of the disease?

Uncontrolled movement called chorea, behavioral changes. Muscle rigidity is noted. Impaired gait. Impaired judgement and cognition are common.

What age is most affected?

30 to 50 years old.

Is there a cure?

No, the disease will get progressively worse.

Clinical Priorities

1. The client with Huntington's disease may experience memory loss.

2. Violent outbursts may be a part of the behavioral changes and mood swings.

3. The time from the first symptom to the death of the client is 10-30 years.

4. This condition is often confused with Parkinson's disease which also has rigidity and slow movement. However, clients with Parkinson's disease do not have the cognitive impairment seen in Huntington's disease.

Immunizations

What vaccine is given at each age?

Birth	Hep B #1
2 months	Hep B #2, DTap, Hib, IPV, PCV
4 months	All 2-month immunizations except Hep B
6 months	All 2-month immunizations
12 months	MMR #1, Hib, PCV, varicella

*some resources say Hep B #2 can be given at 1 month.

Tetanus and diphtheria are optional vaccinations; what is the earliest age they can be given?

2 months

What is a booster shot?

An additional dose of the vaccination to increase effectiveness.

What are the side effects of vaccines?

Low-grade fever, tenderness, swelling at the site, children may become irritable.

What medication should be given for these effects?

Acetaminophen

Never give _____ to children experiencing these effects.

Aspirin

41

When should the meningitis vaccination be given?

Before a client goes to college

If an adult woman receives an MMR shot, what should you teach her?

Wait three months before trying to become pregnant. 2 doses of the vaccine should be given 28 days apart.

How soon can a child get the influenza vaccination?

Not until six months

Do not give MMR or the chickenpox vaccine to clients allergic to what?

Neomycin

What is active immunity?

Stimulating the body to produce antibodies by giving the client a vaccine.

What is passive immunity?

Antibodies that are formed in another body but passed down to another person for short-term use. Examples: When a baby gets their mother's antibodies through the placenta or breast milk.

	Active Immunity	Passive Immunity
How is immunity acquired?	The patient has responded to an antigen and produced his/her own antibodies.	The patient is given antibodies by someone else.
Types	Natural-infection Artificial- induced by vaccines	Natural-transfer of maternal antibodies Artificial-injection of immunoglobulines
Time Advantage	Immediate immunity	Immunity effective only after lag time.

Clinical Priorities

1. Let's discuss the difference between a vaccination and immunization. Vaccination: The *act* of introducing a vaccine into the body to produce protection from a specific disease. Immunization: The *process* by which a person becomes protected against a disease. There are different ways a patient can receive an immunization. For example, contracting chicken pox and recovering from it allows the client to develop immunity. Receiving a vaccine is another process to immunity.

2. Clients allergic to gelatin should be educated that some vaccines contain the ingredient.

3. Anaphylaxis is a potential life-threatening adverse reaction to vaccines.

4. Human papillomavirus (HPV) vaccine should be given to adolescents before they become sexually active.

Inflammatory Bowel Disease

Two primary types

	Crohn's Disease	Ulcerative Colitis
Location of disease	Anywhere in the digestive tract from the mouth to anus	Primarily in the colon
Signs	3-4 semi-soft stools, diarrhea. No blood will be present Anorexia, Fistulas	Bloody diarrhea Lower abdominal cramps Weight loss Anemia may be present due to bleeding.
Lifestyle	Associated with smoking High risk for malnutrition, malabsorption	Associated with non-smokers
Treatment	Anti-inflammatory aminosalicylates Glucocorticoids NPO Status with bowel rest during flares Small frequent meals avoiding dairy and greasy foods. Low fiber will help relieve diarrhea. Surgery will not help; disease will continue to come back in other areas of the digestive system.	Anti-inflammatory steriods NPO Status with bowel rest during flare ups. Clients should limit intake of caffeine. Sigmoidoscopy is key for diagnosis. This condition is managed surgically to remove the affected area.

Incentive Spirometry

Incentive spirometry is a method of ___ ___ that helps maximize lung inflation.

Deep breathing

Instruct the client to place _____ tightly around the mouthpiece.

Lips

As the client is breathing slowly and deeply which direction should the ball or piston travel?

To the top of the chamber

Incentive spirometry is used after surgery to prevent_____.

Atelectasis and pneumonia

Clinical Priorities	1. The nurse should monitor the lung sounds for improvement.
	2. The client should be instructed to hold their breath for 3-5 seconds.
	3. Incentive spirometry is performed with a device called an *incentive spirometer*.
	4. Clients in pain or those with dementia might be unable to perform incentive spirometry exercises.
	5. The client should do incentive spirometry 5-10 times per hour while awake.
	6. The best position is sitting up as erect as possible, ideally high-Fowler's position.

Increased Intracranial Pressure (ICP)

What is the normal intracranial pressure range?	5-15 mm Hg
What are the common causes of ICP?	Trauma, hemorrhage, edema and tumors
What should the nurse assess?	The level of consciousness (It will decrease as the intracranial pressure increases.)
What is the earliest sign of ICP?	Decreased level of consciousness
The adult client will often appear?	Restless, agitated, reporting headaches.
What are the signs of ICP in babies?	Bulging fontanelles strabismus, vomiting, seizures, high pitched cry, lethargy.
Client may report _____.	Projectile vomiting without nausea
How will the vital signs appear with ICP?	Blood pressure (up) Temperature (up) Respiration (up then down) Heart rate (up)
What is widening pulse pressure and how is it related?	When systolic blood pressure goes up and diastolic pressure continues to go down so that they become further apart (e.g., 135/40 is a bad sign!) A widening pulse pressure indicates deteriorating cardiovascular health.
What is Cushing's Triad?	Three things: widening pulse pressure, Cheyne stokes respirations, and bradycardia.
Initiate _____ precautions.	Seizure
What are the late signs of ICP?	Unilateral pupil dilation, hypertension or hypotension bradycardia
Elevate the head of the bed to?	10 to 30 degrees, to promote jugular venous outflow.

Which medications will be prescribed?	Anticonvulsants Antihypertensives Corticosteroids Diuretics
Teach the client not to ____, ___, or _____.	Strain, cough, or sneeze as these actions can increase ICP.
Nursing interventions would be to?	Decrease environmental stimuli. Maintain body temperature. Limit fluid intake. Monitor intake and output.

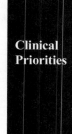

Clinical Priorities

1. The immediate action is to establish a baseline neurological status, this will help determine further deterioration.

2. The <u>cerebral metabolic rate</u> increases with elevated body temperature, so it is important for the nurse to monitor the patient's temperature.

3. Seizure precautions include decreasing environmental stimuli: dim lights, reduced noise, suction and oxygen at the bedside.

4. Do not give meperidine hcl as it will increase intracranial pressure.

Instillation of Ear Medications

The medication should be _____ temperature?	Room - too hot or cold will have side effects (nausea, dizziness etc)
Which position should the client be placed in when receiving ear medication?	Supine, with affected ear up
When administering ear meds to an adult, draw the pinna back and _____.	Up
When administering ear meds to a child, draw the pinna back and _____.	Down
How many minutes should the head be be tilted to allow medication to travel through the ear canal?	5 minutes

Clinical Priorities

1. All ear drops should be a sterile solution in case the ear drum is ruptured.

2. The nurse should wear non-sterile gloves.

3. Pulling the pinna straightens the ear canal.

4. Avoid touching the ear with the dropper tip as with will contaminate the dropper and the medication inside of the bottle.

5. Drops should be placed on the side of the ear canal. Placing drops directly in the canal on the tympanic membrane will cause the patient discomfort.

6. Cotton balls should only be placed in the ear after medication administration if there is an order by the doctor.

Instillation of Eye Medications

When giving eye medications, do this to prevent medication from going into the lacrimal duct.

Apply pressure to the inner canthus.

Pull the _____ eye lid down against the _____.

Lower, cheek

Squeeze the drop in the _____.

Conjunctiva sac

If more than one drop is prescribed, wait ___ to ___ minutes before applying another drop.

3 to 5 minutes

Do not let the _____ touch the ____.

Medication bottle, eyeball

Clinical Priorities	1. The eye is the most sensitive organ to which medication may be applied to.
	2. The cornea is especially sensitive; all medication should be placed in the conjunctival sac.
	3. The nurse should wear non- sterile gloves.
	4. The head should be tilted back to apply eye drops unless the patient has a cervical spine injury.

Intravenous Therapy

Why are IV fluids used?

They are a quick way to replace nutrients, water, and electrolytes

What are the three types of IV fluid?

Isotonic, hypotonic, and hypertonic.

Describe isotonic fluid and give examples.

Isotonic fluids have a similar concentration to blood. This is important because the fluids will not cause water to move in or out of the cell. The size of the cell remains normal. Examples are: 0.9% normal saline, Lactated ringer, 5% Dextrose in Water (D5W)

Why would the nurse give isotonic fluids?

In conditions such as diabetic ketoacidosis, burns- to replace sodium and chloride. And 0.9 % normal saline is always hung with blood**

Describe hypotonic fluids and give examples.

A hypotonic fluid is less concentrated than the blood. This would cause water to move into the cell. The size of the cell will swell or increase. Examples are: 0.45% normal saline, 0.33% normal saline, 2.5% Dextrose water.

Hypotonic fluids should not be given for which conditions?	Patients with increased intracranial pressure, trauma, and skin burns as hypotonic fluids will cause the cells to swell and create further damage. Also hypotension as it lowers the blood volume.
Why would the nurse give hypotonic fluids?	In conditions such as dehydration, hypernatremia; and if the patient needed their blood pressure to be lowered.
Why should hypotonic fluids be closely monitored?	Because a rapid increase in fluid shifting into the cells can cause cellular and cerebral edema.
Describe hypertonic fluids and give examples.	Hypertonic fluids are more concentrated than the blood. This would cause water movement out of the cell. The size of the cell shrinks. Examples: 5% normal saline 5% dextrose in normal saline, 5% dextrose in Lactated Ringer's 5% dextrose in 0.45% normal saline
Why would the nurse give hypertonic fluids?	In condition such as hypovolemia (low blood pressure) hypertonic solutions can be given to increase blood pressure. Hypertonic solutions can provide sodium and other electrolytes while adding minimal water.
Why should hypertonic fluids be closely monitored?	Because it can cause electrolyte imbalance and dehydration.
Which conditions are contraindicated for hypertonic fluids?	Cellular dehydration, kidney damage, and heart disease.
Before the nurse starts IV fluids the _____ should be assessed.	Intravenous (IV) site

Clinical Priorities

1. An order is needed to initiate any IV fluid.

2. IV fluids can be administered by an IV pump or gravity.

3. IV fluids are typically contraindicated in clients who have renal impairment.

4. Primary infusions usually come in larger volumes (1000 mL, 500 mL) Secondary infusions also referred to as "IV piggyback" are intermittent infusions that are attached to the primary bag. Piggybacks are usually a medication such as an antibiotic.

5. Not all IV fluids and IV medications are compatible. Unwanted particles may develop when incompatible IV fluids and IV medications are mixed. This is a significant health danger to the patient.

Intravenous Complications

	Extravasation	Infiltration	Phlebitis
Definition	The leakage of a vesicant into intravascular tissue.	The leakage of an IV fluid or medication into extravascular tissue. *This medication/fluid is a non-vesicant.*	Inflammation of the vein
Cause	Dislodged catheter Occluded vein	Dislodged catheter Occluded vein	Irritating solutions Rapid infusion rates Prolonged use of the same catheter
Clinical Signs	Pain, redness, swelling, increased skin temperature at the site. Fluid leaking from the IV site. Tight skin and blanching may be noted. *Numbness and tingling, blistering or tissue necrosis. Deep pitting edema and circulatory impairment.	Pain, redness, swelling, increased skin temperature at the site. Fluid leaking from the IV site. Tight skin and blanching may be noted.	Pain, redness, swelling, increased skin temperature at the site.
Nursing Interventions	Stop IV infusion. Elevate the extremity. Prepare antidote if one is available. Monitor and photograph the site. Frequently monitor the site. *Do not remove the IV if it is a vesicant. Leave the catheter in place!	Stop the infusion. Elevate the extremity. Apply a warm compress. Insert a new IV catheter in the opposite extremity.	Stop the infusion. Frequently monitor the site. Apply a warm compress. Insert a new IV access in the opposite extremity.

Clinical Priorities	1. Common IV vesicants: diazepam, dopamine, calcium chloride, potassium in high doses. (Do not memorize this list, just know many medications are vesicants.) 2. Secure all IV catheters with transparent tape to enable proper site assessment.

Laminectomy

Surgery is the removal of _____ so the spinal cord can be seen.   Bone

To move the client after surgery, _____ this client!   Log roll

What position must the client remain in?   Flat

The client is at risk for which type of infection?   Arachnoiditis

Clinical Priorities	1. To ensure healing the spinal column must remain in alignment, this requires the client to rest and eat in the flat position. 2. A fracture bedpan will allow the client to remain flat which using the bathroom. 3. Monitor for signs of nerve root compression by asking the client to leg strength, ability to wiggle the toes, and ability to detect touch.

Lead Poisoning

What is the highest risk factor of ingesting lead?	Age: younger kids put things in their mouths.
What item is most likely to cause lead poisoning?	Lead paint chips
The most dangerous side effect of children ingesting lead is _____.	Developmental disability
What are the clinical signs of lead lead poisoning?	Headache, abdominal pain, fatigue, muscle weakness and respiratory depression. Increased clinical signs are based on the dose.
How is lead poisoning treated?	Chelating agents
How are the chelating agents given?	By receiving many IM injections.
Do not give _____ to induce vomiting.	Ipecac syrup

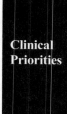

Clinical Priorities

1. Ipecac syrup is no longer recommended due to parents incorrectly administering the medication. Heart problems can develop if improperly used.

2. Iron and calcium help to reduce the levels of lead in the body.

3. Chelating agents

   Dimercaprol, administered IV, give in first 12-24 hrs. Peanut allergy is contraindicated.

   Ethylenediaminetetraacetic acid (CaNa$_2$ EDTA), given IV with dimercaprol or given IM with lidocaine to reduce pain.

Legal Issues

Negligence is when a nurse does _____.	Not provide appropriate care according to set standards
If a nurse does a treatment without consent, it is example of _____?	Battery
If the client falls out of bed because the nurse forgot to put up the side rails, this is considered?	Neglect
Any nursing action that has the word "threat" should be considered an _____.	Assault
Advanced directives are important because they_____.	Allow the client to direct how and what care they want to receive if they become unable to make decisions in the future.
Are advanced directives mandatory for a client?	No-they are optional.

The document that specifically names a person decisions on another person's behalf is a _____.

durable power of attorney make

The client must be of _____ to write a will.

sound mind

Clinical Priorities	1. Patient confidentiality is a right protected by the Health Insurance Portability and Accountability Act (HIPAA).
	2. Anytime a nurse shares medical information with anyone other than the patient he or she must have written permission to do so.
	3. Information can be share with parents of a patient until they turn 18. There are a few exceptions to this rule such as: minor child seeks birth control, an abortion, or becomes pregnant.
	4. A nurse should not take photos or videos of patient on personal devices or cellphones.

Lung Sounds

What is the cause of crackles?

Fluid or secretions in the airway

When would the nurse hear crackles?

On inspiration

What are some possible causes of crackles?

Pneumonia, edema, or bronchitis.

What is another name for crackles?

Rales

What are the characteristics of wheezes?

High-pitched musical sounds

When would the nurse hear wheezes?

On inspiration and expiration

What are the possible causes of wheezing?

Asthma, smoking, allergic reactions

Wheezes can often be heard without a _____.

Stethoscope

_____ air will help relieve symptoms of wheezing.

Humidified

What are the characteristic of stridor?

A high-pitched harsh sound heard in *UPPER* airway

What are the causes of stridor?

Laryngeal spasm, swelling, croup and epiglottitis

Stridor is often confused with _____.

Wheezing

In which age group is stridor often seen?

Children

Clinical Priorities	1. The vital signs may be delegated to the unlicensed assistive personnel.
	2. The normal respiratory rate for an adult is 12-20 breaths per minute at rest, the normal oxygen saturation of the blood is 94-98%.
	3. Anteroposterior-transverse ratio should be 1:2. A patient with a 1:1 ratio is barrel-chested.
	4. The nurse should listen to lung sounds from side to side rather than down one side then the other side. This side-to-side pattern allows the nurse to compare sounds in symmetrical lung fields.
	5. The diaphragm of the stethoscope is the larger flat side that is used to hear normal and high-pitched sounds that occur in the lungs.

Lyme Disease

This type of infection is caused by?

Bite from a tick

What are the clinical symptoms?

Fever, chills, and the bull's eye rash.

How long after a bite can you test for this disease?

Between 4 to 6 weeks

What is the treatment plan?

Take antibiotics:
DOXYCYCYLINE (Adults)
AMOXICILLIN   (Children)

Clinical Priorities

1. Instruct patients to remove the tick as soon as it is found making sure to remove the head of the tick not just the body protrusion.

2. With early treatment most patients recover rapidly.

ReMar NCLEX Planner Page	
Name:	**Date:**

Lessoned I have learned while studying:
1.
2.
3.

Is studying for NCLEX still my top priority? Why or why not?

What actions will I take to ensure my week is productive?
1.
2.
3.

This week I am looking forward to:

Today I am grateful for:

What you do today WILL change all of your tomorrows!

Maslow's Hierarchy of Needs

What are the most important factors in order?

Physiological Needs
Safety and Security
Love and Belonging
Self-Esteem
Self-Actualization

Mastectomy

This surgery is to remove _____ tissue or the _____.

Breast tissue or nipple

After surgery,_____ the affected arm to prevent_____.

Elevate, lymphedema

No _____ _____or _____ in the affected arm.

Blood pressure, venipuncture

Always assess the site for signs of _____ after surgery.

Infection

List signs of clinical site infection.

Swelling, redness, fever, chills, elevated WBC count

Clinical Priorities

1. Consider the following terms for memorization: Lumpectomy- A surgery to remove cancerous tissue from the breast. This is considered a breast saving surgery. Mastectomy- A surgery to remove the breast. Mammoplasty-A surgery to reconstruct the breast.

2. The patient should be instructed to not carry packages, handbags, or luggage with the affected arm. Also avoid blood pressure cuffs, and intravenous injections all of these are recommended to avoid developing cellulitis and breast cancer related lymphedema.

Medication Administration

What are the six rights of medication administration?

Right: Client, Medication, Documentation, Dose, Time and Route

What two verifiers can a client give before the nurse administers the medication?

Name and birthdate

Do not store medications _____.

At the bedside

Can the nurse give medication prepared by another RN?

No, never do this! It is illegal.

What does it mean if a medication is PRN?

It means give when needed

Do not _____ sustained-release capsules or enteric-coated tablets.

Crush

What should a nurse do if she/he administers the wrong medication?

Notify physician; DO NOT document in client's chart and complete an incident form. This is not part of client records

Clinical Priorities

1. Always ask patient about allergies, types of reactions, and severity of reactions.

2. All medications require an assessment before administration.

3. If a patient questions a medication the nurse should not administer the medication but contact the healthcare provider.

Meniere's Syndrome

What is it?	Meniere's disease is an inner ear disorder.
What are the symptoms?	Tinnitus, unilateral hearing loss, and dizziness
What are the causes?	Viral and bacterial infections and allergic reactions.
Describe Meniere's attacks.	It results in severe, sudden attacks that may cause permanent hearing loss. Nausea and vomiting can also be present.
What is the best environment for a client with this disease?	Bed rest in a quiet room, sedatives can be given to keep client calm. Low-playing music helps with the tinnitus. The client should move the head and ambulate slowly.
What should the client's diet be?	Low sodium to help reduce fluid overload in the ear.
Is surgery needed?	In severe cases a removal of the labyrinth (or labyrinthectomy) is performed.

Clinical Priorities

1. Meniere's disease usually starts in one ear but later may involve both.

2. Smoking, infections, and a high salt diet may worsen the disease.

3. Patients can be treated with diuretic medications such as hydrochlorothiazide or acetazolamide.

Meningitis

What is meningitis?	Inflammation of arachnoid and pia mater of the brain and spinal cord
How is it transmitted?	Direct contact and droplet
What are the signs and symptoms?	Nuchal rigidity, tachycardia, headache, nausea, and vomiting.
Meningitis can also cause _____.	increased intracranial pressure

What two physical signs are positive?	Positive Kernig's and Brudzinski sign
What are the nursing interventions?	Monitor LOC, vital signs, initiate seizure precautions, maintain droplet isolation, and elevate the head of the bed.
What medications are prescribed?	Antibiotics and analgesics

Clinical Priorities

1. There are two types of meningitis bacterial and viral. The viral type does not require antibiotics or isolation precautions.

2. The lumbar puncture is done by collecting cerebrospinal fluid to check for signs meningitis.

3. The nurse should assess the patient's vital signs and neurological status at least every 4 hours.

4. Osmotic diuretics may be prescribed to reduce cerebral edema.

Mongolian Spots

What do these spots look like?	Bluish-black spots on body
Where can you find these spots?	On the back and buttocks of newborns
In which race are these spots mostly seen?	Asian and African Americans
Are they harmful and how long do they appear?	No. They are normal in newborns and they gradually fade over time.

Clinical Priorities

1. Mongolian spots are typically 2-8 cms wide. They have irregular shape without defined edges.

2. Mongolian spots are not cancerous and do not require any kind of treatment.

3. If the spots persist beyond teenage years and into adulthood, removal procedures are available.

Multiple Sclerosis (MS)

True or false? MS is a chronic, progressive degenerative disease of the nervous system.	True
What part of the nervous system is affected?	The problem is with demyelinization of the white matter of the brain and spinal cord.
Is there a cure for MS?	No
What are the signs of MS?	Muscle spasms, weakness, Bowel & bladder dysfunction numbness in the extremities, and visual disturbances.
Which medication will be given for spasms?	Baclofen

What medication will be given to reduce the amount of time a client experiences exacerbated symptoms?

Corticosteroids

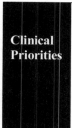

Clinical Priorities

1. The age of onset is 20-40 years of age.

2. The condition affects women more than men. Caucasian people more than any other race.

3. It is expected for the client to use mobility aids to improve unsteady gait.

4. The nurse should allow the client to remain as independent as possible.

5. Physical and speech therapy should be a part of the treatment regimen.

Munchausen Syndrome

What is the definition of this syndrome?

A psychiatric disorder that causes a person to self-inflict injury to his/her own body. The person may also say that he/she has a mental disorder. This is all done to get attention from healthcare workers.

What is Munchausen syndrome by proxy (MSBP)?

An individual, typically a mother, intentionally causes or makes up an illness in a child under their care for attention.

Clinical observations

The child will have issues with no explained etiology. Treatment of the issue does not stop the child from needing hospital visits. Assessments indicates the child is healthy, symptoms get better when child is away from the caregiver.

Nurse priority: Protect the child!

Clinical Priorities

1. MSBP is a type of child abuse and can result in long-term harm and even death.

2. The commonly reported medical conditions used are apnea, anorexia, diarrhea, seizures, and pain.

3. All forms of child abuse are mandatory to report.

Myasthenia Gravis

True or false? Myasthenia gravis is an autoimmune disease that results in extreme fatigue and muscle weakness.	True
What is the malfunction in the body?	The body produces antibodies that block acetylcholine receptors
Is there a cure for myasthenia gravis?	No
What are the clinical signs?	Difficulty talking, chewing, weak eye muscles, visual disturbances, and unsteady gait.
Will the symptoms of myasthenia gravis worsen with activity?	Yes, they will.
The _____ test is performed to diagnosis myasthenia gravis.	Tensilon
If the client's muscle strength is increased, the test is _____ for myasthenia gravis.	Positive
What medication will be given?	Anticholinesterase Plasmapheresis is also a possible treatment too.

Clinical Priorities	1. The client should take their medications 30 minutes before eating.
	2. The client should avoid factors that may precipitate a myasthenia crisis such as: stress, surgery, use of streptomycin.
	3. Be alert of signs of myasthenia crisis: sudden inability to swallow, speak, or maintain a patient airway.

Myocardial Infarction (MI)

What is the cause of an MI?	A decreased oxygen supply to heart
Where is the pain felt?	Substernal (sudden, crushing, radiating to jaw, shoulders, back) & lasting longer than 30 minutes.
MI pain is not relieved by _____ or _____.	Rest or nitroglycerin
What changes would you see on an EKG?	ST elevation inverted T waves
What lab values will be elevated?	CK-MB CPK Troponin LDH WBC

Which medications are given for an MI?	**M.O.N.A.** **M**orphine, **O**2, **N**itroglycerin, **A**spirin
In which order should MONA be administered?	Oxygen, nitroglycerin, Aspirin, morphine O.N.A.M.
What activity is prescribed for this client?	Bed rest
What is angina pectoris?	Chest pain due to the heart not receiving enough oxygen
Where is the pain located?	The same area of the chest as reported in an MI.
What are some common causes of angina?	Early-morning activity Eating large meals, general stress, exercise, and smoking
How is stable angina different from an MI?	Angina is chest pain that has a typical onset location, lasts for three to five minutes and is relieved by nitroglycerin or rest.
What is unstable angina?	It is chest pain that occurs while the client is resting.
Which diagnostic tests are utilized?	A cardiac catheterization, A coronary artery bypass An exercise stress test EKG with no ST elevation indicates angina instead of a MI.

Clinical Priorities

1. The primary goal of acute management is to rapidly restore blood flow to the acutely occluded coronary artery.

2. Supplemental oxygen delivery needed for ischemia management is given via *nasal cannula* at 2-4 LPM.

3. Beta blockers can also be given to prevent dysrhythmias.

Neomycin Sulfate

What is it?	It's an aminoglycoside that reduces the number of bacteria in the colon
Why does this matter?	It's used for GI tract before surgery
How is it used in clients with hepatic encephalopathy?	It can be used when ammonia levels are elevated in the liver.

Clinical Priorities

1. Aminoglycosides can cause fetal harm to pregnant women.
2. The oral form of neomycin may result in the overgrowth of fungi.
3. Aminoglycosides should be used in caution with patients with myasthenia gravis or parkinsonism.
4. Patients should not take antibacterial medications to treat viral infections.

Neuroleptic Malignant Syndrome (NMS)

When does this syndrome occur?

It could occur any time a client is on anti-psychotic medication; it is most common when the treatment begins or if doses are increased.

What are the signs of N.M.S.?

Tachycardia – extreme fever, altered LOC, seizures, muscle rigidity, elevated lab values (e.g., WBC and LFT)

What is the treatment?

Discontinue the medication. Initiate safety and seizure precautions. Give antipyretics to reduce fever.

Clinical Priorities	1. The client will present in a catatonia-like state, there will be extrapyramidal signs.
	2. The primary goal of NMS treatment is to manage stiffness and hyperthermia while preventing severe complications.
	3. Severe complications include: respiratory failure, rhabdomyolysis, and renal failure.

Nasogastric (NG) Tube

What position should the client be in during NG tube placement?

High Fowler's with head tilted forward

The NG tube goes from the ___ to ____.

Nose to stomach

What is a Salem sump?

Double lumen of NG tube used to decompress the stomach

What are the measuring points for process determining the length of insertion?

Nose to earlobe to xiphoid

If the client starts to gag during placement should the nurse continue the procedure?

Yes, wait for client to stop gagging or coughing, then continue to advance; offer water to help the tube go down.

What should be done before using the NG tube for the first time?

X-ray, aspirate for gastric content (pH should be less than 4)

If the NG tube is to suction, should the nurse turn off the suction when medications are given orally?	Yes, for at least 30 minutes
If a client vomits during the procedure should the nurse keep going with the NG tube?	Yes, wait for a few minutes, then proceed. Let the client know that they will feel better once the NG tube is in place.

Clinical Priorities

1. Conditions that contraindicate an NG tube are: facial trauma, deviated, or swollen nasal septum.

2. Nebulized lidocaine has been shown to relieve discomfort during procedure.

3. Because the dominant hand will be used to insert the tube the nurse should stand on the client's right side if right-handed or left side if left-handed.

4. A water soluble lubricant should be used at the proximal tip.

5. The nurse and client should identify a hand signal before the procedure to communicate.

Nitroglycerin

What is the action of nitroglycerin?	Systemic and coronary vasodilation
What conditions are treated by nitroglycerin?	Angina, cocaine abuse, it can be given before activities that cause chest pain.
If nitroglycerin is given sublingually for angina pain and it is not relieved, what should the nurse do?	Give an additional tablet in five minutes. Up to three tablets can be taken over 15 minutes. The patient should call 911 after the first dose.
If nitroglycerin is given SL and the client reports a stinging sensation, is that normal?	Yes, it means the tablet is fresh.
What is the most common side effect reported?	Headache
What are other common side effects?	Hypotension, tachycardia, dizziness, and syncope
If a client has on a transdermal ointment or nitroglycerin patch, should the nurse rotate sites during application?	Yes, to prevent skin irritation.
Do not place a nitroglycerin patch over a _____.	Pacemaker
The client's nitroglycerin patch should be removed before having a _____ scan.	MRI
Should a client take nitroglycerin prophylactically before sex?	Yes, to prevent chest pain

If a male client is taking sildenafil, what should the nurse tell him?

Don't take with nitroglycerin

IV nitroglycerin and all IV dysrhythmics should be placed on an _____.

Infusion pump

What is verapamil used for?

To treat blood pressure and angina

Clinical Priorities	1. The client should not eat or drink while taking nitroglycerin sublingual.
	2. To prevent angina the client should take 1 tablet 5-10 minutes before the activity.
	3. The tablet can be placed under the tongue, or also between the cheek and the gum.

NSAIDs

What does it stand for?

Nonsteroidal Anti-Inflammatory Drugs

What type of drugs are they?

Aspirin and Aspirin-like drugs

What do NSAIDs do?

Reduce pain and body temperature and inhibit platelet and inhibit platelet aggregation.

Clients should take NSAIDs with a full glass of ___ or _____ to prevent stomach irritation.

Water, milk

Aspirin toxicity will cause _____ in the ears.

Tinnitus

Teach clients to avoid _____ when taking NSAIDs to decrease stomach irritation.

Alcohol

NSAIDs increase/decrease bleeding potential.

Increase

How soon should a client stop taking NSAIDs before having surgery?

1 week

Kids shouldn't take NSAIDs when they have flu-like symptoms due to the risk of?

Reye's syndrome

Nursing success means different things to each one of us. Your journey is unique in that only you can determine how far you go. Build a life you are proud to live!

Nursing Mnemonics

"A.D.P.I.E." for **The Nursing Process**
    Assessment
    Diagnosis
    Planning
    Implementation
    Evaluation

"H.E.L.L.P" for **Pre-eclampsia Syndrome (Severe)**
    Hemolysis
    Elevated
    Liver
    Low
    Platelet Count

"L.I.O.N" for **Maternal Fetal Distress**
    Left Side
    Initiate IV Fluids
    Oxygen via Face Mask
    Notify the doctor

P.A.L.S.Y." for **Cerebral Palsy Features**
    Paresis
    Ataxia
    Lagging motor development
    Spasticity
    Young

"S.M.A.R.T" for **Parkinson's Disease**
    Shuffling gait
    Mask – like face
    Akinesia
    Rigidity
    Tremor

"A.S.T.H.M.A" for **Asthma Medications**
    Adrenergics (Beta 2 Agonists Albuterol)
    Steroids
    Theophylline
    Hydration (IV)
    Mask O_2
    Anticholinergics

"It's Not My Time" **Pre-Term Labor Drugs**
    Indomethacin (NSAID)
    Nifedipine (C.C.B.)
    Magnesium sulfate
    Terbutaline

"M.O.N.A" for **(MI) Medications**
    Morphine
    Oxygen
    Nitrogen
    Aspirin

"R.N." (R then N) for **Drawing Mixed Insulin**
    Air into NPH
    Air into Regular
    Draw up **R**egular, then
    Draw up **NPH**

"S.T.R.I.P.E." TB antibiotics
    ST-reptomycin
    R-ifampin
    I-soniazid
    P-yrizinamide
    E-thambutol

To describe fetal heart rates, remember VEAL CHOP

Variable Decelerations	=	**C**ord Compression
Early Decelerations	=	**H**ead Compression
Accelerations	=	**O**xygenation is ok
Late Decelerations	=	**P**lacental Insufficiency (bad sign)

Note: There are literally hundreds of mnemonic word tools out there! When learning mnemonics, be careful not to go overboard requiring you to remember multiple things in addition to the nursing content. Since we like to get straight to the point I've identified the most common for NCLEX.

Obstetrics History

What is GTPAL?

An acronym to remember essential information in an obstetric history.

What do the letters stand for?

Gravidity, term, preterm, abortion, and living.

What does the gravidity number mean?

It is the number of times a woman has been pregnant, including the current pregnancy.

What does the term number mean?

It is how many full term births a patient has had. This is an infant born after 37-weeks.

What does the preterm number mean?

It is the number of births where the age of the infant is from greater than 20 to 36.6 weeks.

What does the abortion number mean?

It is a general term meaning a pregnancy that has ended without a live birth. An abortion can be induced or spontaneous.

What does the living number mean?

This number represents how many living children the patient currently has.

Clinical Priorities	1. The first prenatal visit should establish dangers to the current pregnancy. The nurse should determine if the client is at risk for STDs, which birth control method if any were used, and if there is currently any spotting.
	2. A urine specimen should be obtained before the patient undresses for the pelvic examination. The patient should empty the bladder so that they are more comfortable during the pelvic examination. It is easier to evaluate the size of the uterus with an empty bladder.

Organ Donation

What do you need to know?

Transplants work best when the donor is living. The organs are matched by blood and tissue type. All organ donations must be put in writing. The living client can their mind about donating their organs up until the time the organ is removed.

Can a nurse approach client or family about donation?

No, only an authorized representative.

Clinical Priorities

1. The assessment of the nurse may be required to identify clients who would make good candidates for organ donation.

2. Organs from deceased donors can only be harvested after brain death or cardiac death.

Orthostatic Hypotension

What is it?

Systolic or diastolic BP drops more than 10 mm Hg and heart rate increases by 10-20 when the client changes position (lying, sitting, and standing) *The blood pressure will go down and the heart rate will go up.*

How will client feel?

Dizzy, light-headed, unsteady

How to assess for orthostatic hypotension?

The nurse should check the blood pressure while client is lying down, sitting up, and standing. Wait five minutes between measurements.

What is the treatment?

IV fluids for volume replacement

Clinical Priorities

1. Patients with orthostatic hypotension have an increased risk of falling or fainting.

2. Orthostatic hypotension occurs more frequently in the morning. The blood pressure is the lowest in the morning.

3. Medications that can cause orthostatic hypotension are: diuretics, antidepressants, and vasodilators.

Osteoarthritis

What is osteoarthritis?	A degenerative disease of the joints
Osteoarthritis is the _____ form of arthritis seen in the elderly.	Number one
Which joints in the body are most affected?	Weight-bearing joints - knees, hips, fingers, back
What are the clinical signs of osteoarthritis?	Limited joint mobility, joint pain, joint stiffness
Is the pain from osteoarthritis relieved by activity or rest?	Rest
Hard nodes will develop on the joints of the fingers, creating deformities. What is this called?	Heberden's nodes
What is the primary medication given for pain?	NSAIDs
_____ may be injected into the joints to treat osteoarthritis.	Corticosteroids
What should the nurse teach the client concerning activity?	Stop exercise if pain occurs. Try to lose weight to help take stress off joints. Use hot or cold therapy to help with pain. Assistive devices (canes, braces, etc.) will help with mobility.
What surgery may be required?	Hip and knee replacements

 Clinical Priorities

1. Splinting is beneficial for those with symptomatic osteoarthritis.

2. Clients with mild to moderate osteoarthritis of the knee or hip should participate in a regular exercise program. Examples are a supervised walking program or hydrotherapy classes.

3. Weight reduction reduces the risk of developing symptomatic knee osteoarthritis.

Otitis Media

This is an infection of the _____ ear.	Middle
Why are children more prone to this?	Because their Eustachian tubes are shorter than adults
What are the signs?	Fever, loss of appetite, rolling head from side to side to promote ear drainage.
What is the treatment?	Analgesics and antibiotics

 Clinical Priorities

1. Encourage the mother to breastfeed as it gives the baby natural immunity.

2. Administer pain medication such as acetaminophen or ibuprofen as prescribed.

3. When indicated for a bacterial infection a 10-day course of an antibiotic is given for otitis media.

Oxygen Delivery Systems

What is the range of the flow rate for a nasal cannula?

The flow rate ranges from 1-6 LPM.

Why is the oxygen flow rate for a nasal cannula below 6?

Nares and mucosa dry out when the rate is high.

What are the benefits of using a nasal cannula?

The client can still eat, drink, talk.

How often should the nasal cannula be changed?

Every day

What should be inspected daily due to irritation?

Skin on face, nares, ears

What is the flow rate range for a simple mask?

6-10 LPM

When applying the mask, what must be done?

Make sure it fits properly, covering mouth and nose

Clients wearing a face mask may feel _____.

Claustrophobic

What makes a Venturi mask different from a regular face mask?

It allows the nurse to control how much room air is to be mixed with oxygen.

Always use a Venturi mask for clients with ____.

C.O.P.D. because the specific O_2 concentration should be noted.

A partial rebreather mask looks like a face mask with a _____ _____ attached to it.

Reservoir bag

Like the other forms of oxygen delivery, the partial rebreather allows ___ ___ to mix with _____.

Room air, pure oxygen

The reservoir bag should be inflated when?

At all times. Please note this.

The non-rebreather mask does not allow _____

Room air to be inhaled.

How would you assess to see if the oxygen delivery system is effective?

A pulse oximetry reading, respiration rate and pattern, arterial blood gas.

Do not use _____ for a moisturizer the nares.

Petroleum jelly can set the client's face on fire. Use a water-soluble jelly.

Clinical Priorities

1. When using a nasal cannula, place the prongs into the patient's nares to fit the tubing around the ears.

2. When using a mask, place the mask over the patient's mouth and nose.

3. If using a non-rebreather mask, partially inflate the reservoir bag before applying the mask.

4. Although all medications given in the hospital require a prescription, oxygen therapy may be initiated without a physician order in emergency situations.

5. The biggest limitation of the nasal cannula is that it is easily dislodged.

65

Pacemakers

What is the indication?

To conduct electrical activity and maintain normal heart rate.

Describe client education on pacemakers.

Check pulse daily. Avoid large magnetic fields (MRI, industrial equipment).
Household appliances can be used. for use. Avoid contact sports.
Report signs of dizziness, fatigue, or SOB to the doctor.
Use cellphones on the opposite side of pacemaker

Clinical Priorities	1. Understand the different types of pacemakers *Atrial* - The pacer spikes before the P waves *Demand* - The pacer fires only when the patient needs it. Also called synchronous pacemaker *Ventricular* - The pacer spike is followed by the QRS complex. 2. Pacemakers are most commonly used to treat bradycardia.

Pancreatitis (Acute)

What is the number-one cause of acute pancreatitis?

Alcohol abuse

What are the symptoms of acute pancreatitis?

Abdominal pain, nausea, vomiting, board-like abdomen Skin discoloration (Cullen's and Turner's sign)

Will eating make the pain better or worse?

Worse, especially fatty foods

Which liver enzymes are elevated with pancreatitis?

Lipase and amylase

What are the nursing interventions?

Make the client NPO. An NG tube may be needed to reduce gastric distention, IV fluids to prevent dehydration. The client should be educated on the detrimental effects of alcohol.

How is the pain treated?

Demerol or hydromorphone

Never give this for pain. Why?

Morphine; it was thought to cause spasms in the pancreatic duct and sphincter of Oddi.

Clinical Priorities	1. Pancreatitis is the inflammation of the pancreas. 2. Significant changes in the vital signs that may indicate signs of shock. 3. Removal of the gallbladder may be necessary if gallstones are the cause of pancreatitis. 4. The supine position often increases a patient's pain. 5. Patients with pancreatitis may experience issues with hyperglycemia due to damaged pancreas cells that are unable to release insulin.

Paracentesis

This is an invasive procedure. The client will need an:

Informed consent

This procedure collects fluid from where?

Peritoneal cavity of abdomen

What to do before procedure?

Measure abdomen, weigh the client and take the vital signs. Have the client void to empty bladder before the procedure.

What position should the client be in during during this procedure?

Sitting on edge of bed

What should the nurse do after the procedure?

Monitor the vital signs, measure the fluid collected, apply sterile dressing to the insertion site and monitor for bleeding.
Make sure urine is not bloody.

Clinical Priorities

1. Liver cirrhosis is the most common cause of ascites formation.

2. Absolute contraindications include an acute abdomen issue, the uncooperative patient, and disseminated intravascular coagulopathy.

3. A distended bladder increases the risk for bladder perforation during the procedure. Monitor the client for bloody urine after the paracentesis.

Parkinson's Disease

This disease is caused by a depletion of _____?

Dopamine

What are the signs of Parkinson's disease?

Bradykinesia, tremors in the hands and feet at rest, rigidity, shuffling steps, and loss of balance

Is this disease process fast or slow?

Slow, progressive

What are the nursing interventions?

Assess the neuro status and swallowing ability, assist with ambulation, encourage fluids to prevent dehydration. Recommend a high-calorie & fiber meals with a low-protein diet.

Which medications are prescribed?

Anti-Parkinson's
Anti-cholinergics

When taking anti-cholinergics, clients should increase _____ to avoid _____.

Fiber, constipation

What are the other side effects of anti-cholinergics?

Blurred vision, dry mouth, photophobia, tachycardia

Which medications will be given to replace dopamine?

Levodopa or Carbidopa-levodopa

Do not take dopamine replacement medications with _____ , as this may cause a hypertensive crisis.

MAOIs

Teach clients taking Parkinson's drugs to follow a _____ _____ diet.

Low-protein

What vitamin should be avoided in the diet?

B6, which blocks the Parkinson's medication therapeutic effect.

Clinical Priorities	1. The nurse should assess the neurologic status and the client's ability to chew and swallow.
	2. Clients should avoid using monoamine oxidase inhibitors because they will precipitate hypertensive crisis.
	3. The client with Parkinson's disease can develop bradykinesia, or akinesia, when ambulating promote safety.

Peptic Ulcer Disease

What bacteria is responsible for most peptic ulcers?

H. pylori

Where are most peptic ulcers found?

Gastric and duodenal

When a client has ulcers, what will the vomit look like?

"Coffee ground"

When a client has ulcers, what will the stool look like?

"Black tarry"

What medications should be avoided?

NSAIDs

Is acetaminophen a NSAID?

No

Ulcers	Gastric	Duodenal
Where are the ulcers?	Stomach	Duodenum
Does stomach acid increase?	No, normal production	Yes, increased production
Where does the pain occur?	Mid-epigastric region	Mid-epigastric region
When does the pain occur?	With meals or after eating "starve a gastric ulcer"	On an empty stomach "feed a duodenal ulcer"

What type of medication will be given to decrease gastric acid production in duodenal ulcers?

H2 blockers and proton pump inhibitors

What are medication examples of H2 blockers?

Ranitidine and Cimetidine

What are the medication examples of proton pump inhibitors?

Generic ending in "- zole"
Esomeprazole
Pantoprazole
Omeprazole)

_____ are prescribed to neutralize gastric acid.

Antacids

What should the nurse teach clients with ulcers to avoid?

Smoking and alcohol

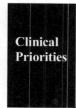

Clinical Priorities

1. The client should avoid the consumption of alcohol or any caffeine containing food.

2. During active bleeding the nurse should assess for hemorrhage, dehydration, and hypovolemic shock.

3. The client should also avoid a diet rich in milk and creams.

4. The client should be instructed to stop smoking as it causes increased acidity in the duodenum.

Peripheral Arterial Disease (PAD)

PAD is an occlusive disease of the _____.

Lower extremities

Will the damage to surrounding tissue occur above or below the arterial occlusion?

Below

Would a pulse be felt in a leg with PAD?

No, it would be absent.

What would the leg look like?

Hairless, cool, pale, with thick toenails.

What is intermittent claudication?

Muscle pain from a decreased blood supply: the pain comes and goes.

The nurse should teach the client not to?

Smoke, wear tight clothing, or apply direct heat to the legs.

The nurse should teach the client to?

Exercise, inspect skin daily, take prescribed medications.

What procedures improve PAD?

Bypass surgery, angioplasty

What does a leg with a venous occlusion look like?

Brown or purple discoloration, edema, or weeping fluid.

Clinical Priorities

1. The PAD is a type of artherosclerosis.

2. Pain worsens when the leg is elevated, the client will feel better when the legs are dangled.

3. PAD is characterized by a slow and progressive narrowing of the arteries.

Pheochromocytoma

A tumor that produces an excessive amount of _____ and _____.

Epinephrine, norepinephrine

This is a problem with the _____ gland.

Adrenal

The clients will experience:

Sustained hypertension, sweating, weight loss, hyperglycemia and headache.

What is the treatment for pheochromocytoma:

Surgical removal of one or both adrenal glands

What will the client need to take after surgery?

Glucocorticoid replacement

Clinical Priorities	1. The nurse should be prepared to collect a 24-hour urine to help diagnose pheochromocytoma.
	2. After an adrenalectomy the nurse should monitor the client for electrolyte imbalance especially potassium levels.
	3. The diet after an adrenalectomy will be a healthy balanced regular diet.

Piaget's Theory of Cognitive Development

Age/Stage	Characteristics
Birth to 2 years - *Sensorimotor*	Child learns about reality by interacting with his/her environment.
2 to 7 years - *Preoperational*	Child moves to pre-logical thinking; learns past, present, future. No abstract yet.
7 to 11 years - *Concrete*	Child moves to logical thinking; able to classify and sort facts. Abstract thinking available. UNDERSTAND DEATH by 10 years old.
11 to adult - *Formal*	Person is able to think and learn as an adult with concrete and abstract reasoning.

Age/Stage	Clinical Priorities
Birth to 2 years - *Sensorimotor*	The child learns through the 5 senses, imitates behaviors, develops object permanence. The beginning of goal-directed actions.
2 to 7 years - *Preoperational*	The child has a one-way logic with the ability to use symbols, egocentrism, children has difficulty with the principle of conservation.
7 to 11 years - *Concrete*	The child uses hands on thinking, understands the need for an identity, and can understand classification.
11 to adult - *Formal*	Person is able to understand scientific reasoning, the nurse is able to explain difficult medical issues. Not all individual reach this stage depending on other medical or psychological factors.

Placenta Previa vs. Abruptio Placenta

What is Abruptio Placenta?

When the placenta detaches itself from the uterine wall

What is Placenta Previa?

The placenta is covering or near cervix, blocking the opening to the vagina.

	Signs	Risk Factors	Dangers	Nursing Interventions
Abruptio Placenta	Sudden, PAINFUL, bleeding with contractions and uterine tenderness	HTN, diabetes, smoking, alcohol (ETOH) abuse, drug abuse	-Decreased oxygen and nutrients to fetus -Premature birth -Blood clots	Bed rest C-section if baby is term Frequent vitals Blood transfusion may be needed so a type and cross of the mother should be ordered.
Placenta Previa	Sudden, PAINLESS, bleeding, bright red in color Usually seen in third trimester	Previous C-section, multiparity, older-age mother	-Maternal hemorrhage -Premature labor	Bed rest C-section if baby is term Frequent vitals Blood transfusion may be needed so a type and cross of the mother should be ordered.

Both conditions will require which three interventions?

Frequent vitals
Fetal ultrasound
Fetal heart monitoring

Which condition has more bleeding?

Placenta previa

Which condition will create a rigid, board-like abdomen?

Abruptio placenta

Abruptio placenta causes which blood clotting disorder?

Disseminated intravascular coagulation (DIC)

If a pregnant client is bleeding vaginally the nurse should avoid a:

A vaginal exam

Clinical Priorities

1. In placenta previa changing the client's position is the priority over oxygenation. The nurse should focus on relieving cord compression.

2. The nurse should assess bleeding, and maintain a perineal pad count for both types of clients.

3. The nurse should observe for shock which is characterized by a rapid pulse, pallor, cold moist skin and a drop in blood pressure.

Plasmapheresis

What is plasmapheresis?

It is removing antibodies that attack the immune system from a client's plasma.

What kind of patients need plasmapheresis?

Client's with systemic lupus erythematosus, multiple sclerosis, Guillain-Barre and other autoimmune diseases.

When plasma is removed what is it replaced by?

Saline or albumin

During plasmapheresis is just the plasma removed?

No whole blood is removed then the plasma is separated.

How long does a plasma exchange take?

1 to 3 hours

What is a potential complication of plasmapheresis?

Hypotension

Clinical Priorities
1. Plasmapheresis can be used in absence of a disease process such as in the case of collecting plasma for donation.
2. Blood is taken out of the body by a large bore needle.
3. During one session of plasmapheresis, 3 to 4 liter of plasma may be removed.
4. Since plasma contains blood clothing factors, the removal may lead to a temporarily decreased ability for the patient's blood to clot.

Pleural Effusion

Pleural effusion is the collection of _____ in the pleural space.

Fluid

What are the signs?

Sharp pain on inspiration tachycardia, shortness of breath with decreased breath sounds

What is the treatment?

Find the cause, monitor breath sounds, performing a thoracentesis.

After a thoracentesis is performed, what may be needed temporarily?

A chest tube to remove residual fluid.

What medication can be prescribed if the fluid is not a large enough amount to perform a thoracentesis?

Diuretic

Clinical Priorities
1. The nurse should monitor the client for breath sounds. Encourage coughing and deep breathing.
2. The client should be placed in a fowler's position.
3. If a pleural effusion is recurrent, prepare the client for pleurectomy or pleurodesis as prescribed.

Polycythemia Vera

What is polycythemia vera?

A disorder of an increased number of erythrocytes, platelets, leukocytes, and the result is thickened blood.

What symptoms will be present?

Headache, SOB, & weakness

On assessment, what is seen?

Purple/red complexion, enlarged spleen, and increased hemoglobin

With polycythemia, will clotting be increased or decreased?

Increased

What is the main treatment?

Phlebotomy (blood draws several times a year)

Clinical Priorities

1. The client should be placed in the semi-fowler's position prior to phlebotomy.

2. Early ambulation and passive leg exercises should be encouraged to prevent thrombotic incidents.

3. The client should be taught not to sit in a crossed legged fashion, place a cushion under the knee, or wear tight clothing.

Post-Traumatic Stress Disorder (PTSD)

What causes PTSD?

Any traumatic event can cause PTSD

What are the signs associated with PTSD?

Nightmare, anxiety attacks sleep disturbances, memory loss, or hypervigilance

These clients will often seem detached. True or false?

True; patients will isolate themselves.

Clients with PTSD are at increased risk for _____.

substance abuse

What is the treatment for PTSD?

Therapy to discuss feelings
Anxiety and depression meds
Support groups

Clinical Priorities

1. Young children may manifest different symptoms. They may wet the bed, forget how to talk or act out a traumatic event during playtime.

2. Cognitive therapy helps patients recognize and modify potentially harmful thinking patterns.

3. Remind the patients that setbacks on the treatment process are not failures but an expected part of the therapy.

Pregnancy Stuff

Rho (D) immune globulin is given to pregnant clients who are Rh _____ but have a Rh____ baby.

Negative, positive

When is Rho (D) immune globulin given?

At 28 weeks' gestation and within 72 hours after delivery It is given twice. This medication prevents the mom from developing antibodies against future Rh positive babies.

Is Rho (D) immune globulin given if the client has a miscarriage?

Yes, if the pregnancy is greater than 13 weeks

Is Rho (D) immune globulin given to the infant?

No, never or to the father

What are tocolytics?

Drugs given to stop preterm labor

What is the mnemonic used to remember the four drugs that can be used for preterm labor?

It's **N**ot **M**y **T**ime

Which medications do the letters stand for?

Indomethacin (NSAID)
Nifedipine (C.C.B.)
Magnesium sulfate
Terbutaline

When giving these medications, what must be monitored continuously?

Fetal heart rate and maternal vital signs

Magnesium sulfate will decrease _____, _____, and _____.

urine output, deep tendon reflexes, and respirations

If a client is given terbutaline, watch for _____.

Tachycardia

Which two drugs are never given to a pregnant client? Think "Two QTs say no to OB's"

Quinolones, Tetracyclines

The umbilical cord in a newborn has _____ arteries and _____ vein.

2, 1

Clinical Priorities	1. As the pregnant woman develops the fetus oxygen consumption increases. This may increase episodes of shortness of breath.
	2. Even if a pregnant client is gaining weight she can still be malnourished. This will present as anemia and small for gestational age baby.
	3. To individualize health, the nurse must first assess the patient's knowledge level about pregnancy expectations.

Presbycusis

This is a form of _____ loss.

Hearing

Is presbycusis a natural process?

Yes

_____ voice tones are hardest to hear.

High

How should the nurse communicate with this client?

Facing towards the patient
The patient should be encouraged to wear a hearing aid.

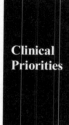

Clinical Priorities

1. The nurse should assess the client's preferred language for verbal and written communication.

2. It is inappropriate to speak loudly, to mumble or slur words.

3. The nurse should instruct the client that cotton-tipped applicators should not be inserted into the ear canal because it can lead to trauma to the canal and can puncture the tympanic membrane.

4. Educate the client on the difficulty of hearing over background noises because sound is coming from all sides. Ask the client to sit with his or her back to the wall so sound is not coming from all sides.

Pressure Ulcers

What are the clinical symptoms of a stage 1 pressure ulcer?

Red, warm, intact skin that doesn't blanche

What is an example of a stage 1 pressure ulcer

It looks like a sunburn

How would you describe a stage 2 pressure ulcer?

Superficial damage to the skin (epidermis or dermis) There will be a break in the skin.

What are some examples of a stage 2 pressure ulcer?

Abrasion, blisters, shallow craters

What is a clinical sign of a stage 3 pressure ulcer?

Skin that is deeply damaged, but does not extend through fascia

What is a clinical sign of a stage 3 pressure ulcer?

Deep crater

What are clinical signs of a stage 4 pressure ulcer?

The skin is deeply damaged, the wound shows muscle tissues and ligaments.

What are some nursing interventions to prevent pressure ulcers from developing?

Turn client every two hours; Keep the skin clean and dry; Encourage proper diet and hydration; Inspect skin and document daily.

Clinical Priorities

1. Inspection of the skin should focus on common pressure points: sacrum, buttocks, heels, the back of the head, elbows, shoulders, hips, and sides of the knees and ankles.

2. Incontinence of urine and feces damage the dermal and epidermal cells.

3. The Braden Scale is an assessment tool used to determine the level of risk a patient has for skin breakdown. Sensory perception, moisture, activity, mobility, friction, and shear are the categories.

Radiation Therapy

What are the types of therapy?

External (outside body)
-Beam and sealed
Internal (inside body)

What are the side effects?

Alopecia, fatigue,
And skin irritation

Clients receiving beam radiation
therapy should wash the area with?

Unscented soap
and water then pat dry

Clients receiving radiation therapy
need private a _____ and _____.

Room, bathroom

No _____ or _____ may come to visit

pregnant women or
small kids

Can a woman with a removed cervical
implant have sexual intercourse?

Yes, 7-10 days after removal.

Clinical Priorities	
	1. The nurse should not apply lotions, powders, ointments to irradiated skin.
	2. There must be a "Caution Radioactive Material" placard taped to the patient's door.
	3. In the event that a patient dies shortly after receiving treatment with radiation implants they must all be removed before the patient's body leaves the floor. The radiation oncologist will remove the implants not the nurse.
	4. Bedding and room wastes should be saved until radioactive sources have been removed and checked. No patient is to leave the hospital without an exit survey by radiation safety.

Raynaud's Disease

What is it?

Vasospasms of the arteries of
the upper & lower extremities

Which body parts are most affected?

Fingers, toes, and cheeks

What does the client feel?

Numbness, tingling, and
swelling; area may feel cold
to the touch.

What are the treatments?

Monitor pulses, vasodilators,
avoid cold and stress, stop
smoking and wear warm clothes.

Clinical Priorities	
	1. The nurse should assess the client for blanching of the extremity, followed by cyanosis from vasoconstriction.
	2. Instruct the client to wear warm clothing, socks, and gloves in cold weather. Advise the client to avoid injuries to fingers and hands due to lack of circulation.
	3. Instruct the client to avoid smoking. Help the client to identify and avoid precipitating factors such as cold and stress.

Retinal Detachment

Will clients experience pain if the retina is detaches?

No, this is painless.

Is this a serious condition?

Yes, this is an emergency.

What are the signs of a detached retina?

Blurred vision, floaters, flashes of light, black spot

What is the treatment for a detached retina?

Surgery to reattach the retina

What are the nursing interventions?

Cover both eyes with patches. No coughing, sneezing, strict bedrest keep head of bed elevated.

Clinical Priorities

1. The nurse should assess the client for flashes of light, floaters or black spots (signs of bleeding), increase in blurred vision, sense of a curtain being drawn over the eyes, and painless loss of central or peripheral vision.

2. The position of the client's head depends on the location of the detachment.

3. The client may wear patches on both eyes to prevent further detachment.

Reye's Syndrome

What is this condition?

Acute encephalopathy (brain disease)

Which other organs are involved?

Liver and kidneys

What is the cause?

Usually, a viral infection There is a link that when aspirin is used to treat a virus Reye's syndrome

What is the treatment?

These patients usually end up in ICU for monitoring and treatment.

Clinical Priorities

1. The condition is most associated with aspirin given for upper respiratory infections, influenza, varicella, or gastroenteritis.

2. Reye's syndrome can also be present by aspirin given following a vaccination again varicella.

3. Salicylates should be avoided for 6 weeks following varicella or the influenza vaccination.

4. The treatment is supportive in nature and the focus is the management of cerebral edema.

Rheumatoid Arthritis

True or false? Rheumatoid arthritis is a chronic systemic inflammatory disease that affects the joints.

True

What are other clinical symptoms associated with rheumatoid arthritis?

Fatigue, weight loss, low-grade fever

Is there a particular age group that is affected?

No, it can occur at any age.

What factor will be found in the blood of a client with this form of arthritis?

Rheumatoid factor

_____ will also be elevated in the blood.

Erythrocyte sedimentation rate

Which joints are mostly affected?

Joints in the hands, wrists, feet, elbows, shoulders

Will these joints be affected unilaterally or bilaterally?

Bilaterally - both hands, feet, and knees, etc.

Due to inflammation of the synovial membranes, which damages cartilage, joint _____ are seen.

Deformities

_____ are the primary drug therapy.

NSAIDS

Should you encourage this client to exercise?

Yes, activity helps with the pain

 Clinical Priorities
1. The disease is characterized by morning stiffness and pain in the affected joints.
2. Early referral to a rheumatologist is critical for accurate diagnosis and prompt implementation.
3. The goal of treatment is to reduce inflammation, pain, preserve function, and prevent deformity.

Scabies

What are the most common symptoms?

Itching and rash

Where is the itching located?

Between the fingers, wrist, around the waist, and genitals. The head and neck are usually affected. Itching is increased at night.

Does a client with scabies require isolation?

Yes, they should be placed under contact isolation.

What is the treatment?

Permethrin 5% Lindane

What nursing education should be included?

Treat all family members at same time. Wash all bed linens in hot water. Itching may occur a few weeks after treatment.

 Clinical Priorities
1. The mode of transmission: physical contact for 15-20 minutes with an infected person. Also, scabies may be acquired by contact by infested bedding.
2. The treatment aims to destroy the scabies mites while also controlling dermatitis for months.
3. Bedding and clothing should be laundered or cleaned and set aside for 14 days in plastic bags.

Seizure Precautions

If the client has a seizure, what is the main goal?	To keep the client safe
True or false? The nurse should mark the time and note client behavior.	True
Should the nurse restrain a client during seizures?	No, do not restrain
What should be done to a client during a seizure?	Turn head to the side, lie the bed flat Pad the head with pillow
Should anything be put in the client's mouth to prevent the client from swallowing his/her tongue?	No, never do this.

Clinical Priorities	1. If the patient is standing or sitting while experiencing a seizure, move them gently to the floor.
	2. Suction and oxygen equipment must be available at the patient's bedside.
	3. Stimulants such as tea, coffee, chocolate, excess salt, spices, and animal proteins trigger seizures by suddenly changing the body's metabolism. Grapefruit and lime juice should be avoided.

Sexually Transmitted Diseases

	Chlamydia	Genital/Oral Herpes	Syphilis
Type of Infection	Bacteria	Virus	Bacteria
Incubation Period	1-3 weeks	3-7 days	Usually, 3 weeks; can range from 9 days to 3 months
Symptoms	Having no signs is common Female: vaginal discharge, lower abdominal pain, burning with urination Male: Urethritis	Urethral discomfort Lesions on vagina Or male genitalia The virus can be transmitted even when no sores are present if the client is shedding the virus.	Primary: chancres Secondary: fever, weight loss, rash
Treatment:	Penicillin	Acyclovir	Doxycycline

	Gonorrhea		Human Papillomar
Type of Infection	Bacteria		Virus
Incubation Period	Men: 3-30 days	Women: 3 to indefinite	3-7 days
Symptoms	Men: urethritis, dysuria, burning yellow or green discharge Female: Yellow discharge, abdominal pain, bleeding with intercourse.		Genital warts on male and female genitalia
Treatment	Penicillin		No cure

Clinical Priorities	1. Sexually transmitted diseases in children should be investigated for sexual abuse.
	2. Clients with HIV should receive the same treatment regimen as those who are HIV negative.
	3. Adults should notify all sexual partners from within 60 days to the onset of symptoms for examination and treatment.
	4. Infected adults should abstain from sex until symptoms are resolved and the partner(s) are tested and treated.

Shingles (Herpes Zoster)

This viral infection is caused by which virus?   Varicella

What are the signs of herpes zoster?   Itching vesicles grouped together
                                                                   on top of a red rash, painful to
                                                                   touch, low-grade fever, malaise

How are shingles spread?   The vesicles contain fluid
                                                                   that transmits the virus.

Where is the rash usually located?   Along a dermatome

What is a dermatome?   An area of skin that gets all
                                                                   of its innervations by a single
                                                                   spinal nerve.

What are some areas of dermatomes?   Face, trunk, back

Will the rash and vesicles be unilateral or bilateral?   Unilateral

What are the isolation precautions for Herpes Zoster?   Respiratory isolation

What is the treatment for shingles?   Analgesics
                                                                   Supportive care
                                                                   Cool compresses
                                                                   Try to keep vesicles intact

What may be seen after the vesicles have healed?   Scarring

Clinical Priorities

1. The vesicles evolve to pustules and then begin to crust over.

2. Shingles is particularly common among clients that are immunosuppressed.

3. Lesions on the tip of the nose, inner corner of the eye indicate involvement of trigeminal nerve.

4. Episodes of herpes zoster generally resolve without intervention.

Sickle Cell Anemia

Is this autosomal trait recessive
or dominant?   Recessive; most commonly
                                                                   seen in African Americans

How is this condition inherited?   A child receives the gene
                                                                   from both parents.

How long do sickled RBCs live
compared to normal RBCs?   6-20 days; normal is 120

What does this put the client at risk for?   Anemia

Whicht test determines sickle cell anemia?   Hemoglobin which shows anemia
                                                                   Sickle testing of blood

The acute exacerbation of sickle cell
anemia is called _____.   Sickle cell crisis or a
                                                                   vaso-occlusive crisis

The most common cause is _____.   Dehydration

This causes the sickled blood to do what?

What is the treatment of a sickle cell crisis?

During a sickle cell crisis, which intervention is done first—give oxygen or hydrate with IV fluids?

Clot

Hydrate with oral and IV fluids Give oxygen to increase tissue perfusion; a blood transfusion may be needed; give pain meds as this is a very painful condition.

Hydrate with IV fluids; remember, during a crisis the blood is clumped together, so the goal is to decrease the viscosity of the blood. Oxygen will not reverse the cause; it will only prevent more clumping.

Clinical Priorities

1. The disorder has its onset during the first year of life. This is a pediatric condition.

2. Chronic hemolytic anemia will produce jaundice, gallstones, and splenomegaly.

3. Upon skin assessment poorly healing ulcers are seen over the lower tibia.

4. Sickle cell anemia may become a chronic multisystem disease with death from organ failure.

Starting an IV

1.	Inform client about procedure and indication.
2.	Gather supplies.
3.	Wash and dry hands.
4.	Use Universal Precautions - wear gloves
5.	Apply tourniquet.
6.	Locate a vein.
7.	Clean the area with alcohol.
8.	Position and insert needle, looking for a flash of blood.
9.	Advance catheter.
10.	Release the tourniquet.
11.	Remove the needle.
12.	Secure the catheter and start IV fluids if ordered.
13.	Document.

Clinical Priorities

1. A written consent is not needed for the specific treatment of IV insertion.

2. The nurse should avoid IV insertion in areas of: fistulas, grafts, active blood clots, burns, edema, or cellulitis.

3. Medication and IV fluids can be given immediately once the nurse clears the site for use.

Sterile Technique

_____ can never be considered sterile, only clean.

Skin

A nurse should never turn the _____ to a sterile field.

Back

If a nurse has on a face mask and sterile gloves, is it okay to adjust the face mask with a gloved hand?

No, because once the gloves touch the mask they are no longer sterile.

A sterile gown is only sterile from the _____ to the ___.

Waist, shoulders

If a sterile wrapper becomes _____ the entire package is no longer sterile.

Wet

Clinical Priorities	1. The nurse should not talk, cough, or sneeze over a sterile field as this leads to contamination.
	2. A sterile field should always be established whenever the nurse intentionally punctures or incises into the body cavity.
	3. If a sterile field is left for any reason, the setup procedure must be restarted.
	4. The goal of starting and maintaining a sterile field is so the client will not get any infections.

Tardive Dyskinesia

What are the clinical signs of Tardive Dyskinesia?

A chewing motion with the mouth, tongue sticking in and out & involuntary movement of the arms and legs.

This is a side effect of which medication?

Antipsychotics

Will the patient have a stiff neck?

Yes

Which class of medication can the nurse give to decrease these effects? I told you earlier.

Anti-Parkinson's

What assessment is used to detect TD?

AIMS exam

Which class of antipsychotic medications have less incidence of TD?

Second generation antipsychotics

Clinical Priorities	1. The first line of management of tardive dyskinesia is to take the client off the antipsychotic medication. This may not be possible in all cases.
	2. Haloperidol is a medication associated with tardive dyskinesia.
	3. Tardive dyskinesia is often confused with Parkinsonism, neuroleptic malignant syndrome and akathisia.
	4. The involuntary movements of tardive dyskinesia can become permanent even after the patient stops taking the medication.

Therapeutic Relationships

Who is involved?

The nurse and client. Client may invite caregivers if necessary

How is a therapeutic relationship different?

A therapeutic relationship only focuses on the needs of the client.

What are the components involved?

Trust, genuine interest, empathy, acceptance, positive regard, self-awareness, and therapeutic use of self

What is positive regard?

A nonjudgmental attitude that implies respect for example calling a client by name and openly and actively listening.

What are the 3 phases of the relationship?

1. Orientation
2. Working
3. Termination

What happens during the orientation phase?

The nurse and client meet
Roles are established
Questions are asked
The nurse discusses termination during this time.

The nurse has to tell the client she must report any harmful or dangerous behavior or comments. This is called a _____ to _____.

Duty to warn

What happens during the working phase?

Problems are identified
Feelings are explored
Goals are set

During the working phase transference can happen with the nurse. What is transference?

Client transfers feelings they have for significant others or parents to the nurse assisting them.

Clinical Priorities

1. The nurse should introduce herself and offer a handshake at the first meeting.

2. The content to be explored is usually determined by the client and the nurse should help facilitate the process.

3. The nurse determines the length of the relationship, the frequency of meetings, and the location.

4. The ending of the nurse client relationship is based on a mutual understanding. However, the client may be ambivalent.

TORCH SYNDROME

What is TORCH?

Toxoplasmosis
Others (Syphillis or Hep B)
Rubella
Cytomegalovirus (CMV)
Herpes simplex

What does TORCH mean in pregnancy?

This is a group of infectious diseases that affect a fetus or newborn baby.

What are the clinical signs?

Difficulty feeding, small areas of bleeding under the skin, small red or purple spots, hepatosplenomegaly.

Are TORCH infections contagious?

Yes they are contagious.

How is TORCH diagnosed?

Through a blood test and viral culture.

How is TORCH treated?

Treatment for TORCH infections depend on the disease. Antibiotics, antivirals, and antiparasitics may be prescribed.

What are the prevention methods to teach?

Avoid contact with the ill. Wash hands often. Do not share drinks or eating utensils. Eat fully cooked meat and eggs. Avoid cleaning cats litter boxes. Wear condom during sex.

Clinical Priorities	1. The is a congenital infection that will be seen at birth, or it can be acquired through breastfeeding.
	2. TORCH infections can cause premature birth, miscarriage, or still birth.
	3. Examples of more "other infections" include: HIV, Zika virus, and chickenpox.

Tracheostomy

What is a tracheostomy?

A surgical procedure that creates an open airway in the trachea

What are the indications for a tracheostomy?

Upper airway obstructions

What is the surgically created opening called?

A stoma

What must the nurse always have at the bedside?

An obturator, a stiff plastic device used for inserting the inner cannula.

Is suctioning a client with a trach a clean or sterile procedure?	Sterile
What should the nurse always do before suctioning a client with a trach?	Hyperoxygenate with 100% oxygen.
Should suction be applied during insertion of the catheter?	No, this can cause damage to the client.
What should the nurse always do after suctioning a client with a trach?	Reoxygenate with 100% O2 2-3 times during inhalation
If a client coughs strongly and the trach becomes dislodged, what are the initial nursing actions?	Keep the airway open by reinserting the obturator, then another inner cannula can be placed. Retention sutures can also be used. Give oxygen if the airway is lost!
If a client is NOT on a ventilator but has a trach, should the inner cuff be inflated?	No, it should be deflated not to block the airway.

Clinical Priorities

1. The surgical opening of the trachea is done below the larynx.

2. A tracheostomy kit is to accompany the patient at all times and this must be checked each shift by the nurse caring for the patient.

3. If a client can speak with a new tracheostomy this is usually an indication that blockage is occurring.

4. Trachea stoma maturation takes approximately 5-7 days after insertion.

5. The air given through a tracheostomy needs to be humidified.

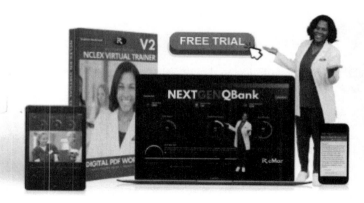

The Transgender Client

How should the nurse address this client?

Ask them what they would like to be called.

If a male completes sexual reassignment surgery will she need a Pap smear exam?

No cervical pap smears are necessary as there will be no cervix in place.

If a female completes sexual reassignment surgery will testicles be formed?

There will be testicles but They will not produce sperm.

Clinical Priorities	1. Transgender clients often avoid medical care. 2. Gender identity is not the same as sexual identity. Gender identity is the patient's internal sense of being a man, woman, or binary. Sexual identity describes the patients romantic physical and emotional attraction for another person. 3. Nurses may have to ask the client if the name on their insurance or other government records match the name that is being currently used. 4. Nurses should also notify the transgender client in advance when they will have to expose their body parts to healthcare workers. This may be a sensitive or difficult act for the client.

Trimethoprim-Sulfamethoxazole

What is this medication used for?

To treat bacterial infections, most commonly UTIs.

What are the contraindications for this medication?

Kidney or liver failure

The severe inflammatory skin disorder can cause

Steven-Johnson syndrome

What are the clinical signs of an allergic to this medication?

Severe skin lesions; blisters; swelling of throat, lips, tongue, fever; headache; rash *lesions can be internally on organs as well

Clinical Priorities	1. The client should be educated on the side effect of increased photosensitivity and will need to use sunscreen and protective clothing. 2. The medication should be taken with a full glass of water. Drinking extra water will help prevent the side effect of crystal in the urine. 3. Agranulocytosis is an expected side effect.

Tuberculosis (TB)

What organism is the cause of TB?

Mycobacterium tuberculosis

What are the signs of active TB?

Productive cough, night sweats, chills, weight loss, low-grade fever

The _____ test is administered by injecting a small amount of tuberculin intradermally.

Mantoux, also called PPD

The Mantoux test is considered positive if the induration (raised skin) is greater than ____ mm.

10

What are the appropriate isolation precautions?

Airborne

The client's negative pressure room should have _____ fresh air exchanges per hour.

6

S.T.R.I.P.E. is the mnemonic for TB antibiotics. What are those medications?

ST-reptomycin
R-ifampin
I-soniazid
P-yrizinamide
E-thambutol

What is the most common side effect of TB antibiotics?

Peripheral neuritis

What are the other side effects?

Muscle ache, GI disturbances, dizziness

What colors will rifampin turn urine, sweat, and tears?

Red or orange

When taking TB antibiotics, which vitamin will be depleted?

B6

Teach the client to avoid _____ to reduce the risk of hepatotoxicity.

Alcohol

Clients taking TB antibiotics are at risk for _____ hepatitis.

Drug-induced

How many consecutive sputum cultures need to be negative for the client to be non-contagious?

3

Clinical Priorities

1. The nurse should use airborne precautions for the client suspected of tuberculosis.

2. The PPD test only indicates exposure to TB it does not confirm the diagnosis.

3. Acid-fast bacilli on a smear of sputum or sputum culture positive for M. tuberculosis is the confirmation.

Ulcerative Colitis

What is the cause of this disease?	The cause is unknown.
What is the pathophysiology?	Inflammatory bowel disease affecting large intestine and rectum
What are the signs or complaints from clients?	Abdominal pain, bloody diarrhea (20 stools/day), nausea, vomiting, and weight loss.
How is ulcerative colitis diagnosed?	Colonoscopy
What are the treatments?	Corticosteroids to reduce inflammation, removal of large intestine and rectum
What will the client need after surgery?	Ileostomy
What is the most appropriate diet for this condition?	Low fiber diet. Teach clients to avoid fiber which increases diarrhea. Fat or greasy foods also to decrease diarrhea. Teach clients to avoid alcohol (ETOH) and caffeine but increase the fluid intake.

Clinical Priorities	1. The stool cultures will be negative for any bacteria or virus.
	2. This condition can cause bleeding which will lead to anemia.
	3. Antidiarrheal agents should not be given in the acute phase of the illness.

von Gierke's Disease

von Gierke's disease is also known as?	Liver glycogen disease
Which age group normally gets this disease?	Children
What are the common clinical signs?	Hepatomegaly, acidosis, hypoglycemia, & delayed growth.
What are the diagnostic tests?	Urine and blood tests, CT
How will the liver appear?	Fatty
What is the treatment plan?	Frequent meals, allopurinol for gout, and a liver transplant.

Clinical Priorities	1. This condition is X-linked and most commonly seen in African black men.
	2. The hepatomegaly will be due to fat and glycogen accumulation.
	3. The nurse should assess the neurological status using the Glasgow Coma Scale as the brain is not receiving adequate amounts of energy.

Wilson's disease

What is Wilson's disease?

It is a genetic defect that causes copper buildup in the body. The body is unable to remove extra copper.

What two organs are affected the most?

Liver and brain

What is the diet for this client?

Low copper

What foods are high in copper and should be avoided?

Lamb, shellfish, vegetable juice, nectarines, dried beans chocolate, and multi-vitamins.

Clinical Priorities

1. This client will need to take a zinc supplement as zinc interferes with the intestinal absorption of cooper.

2. Penicillamine is recommended. *This is not penicillin at all.* This is a chelating agent used for heavy metal toxicity.

3. Hemolysis (destruction of red blood cells) occurs commonly in those with a severe liver disease.

Xtra Stuff

How should the nurse provide cultural care?

Avoid being judgmental. Do not make assumptions. Apologize for cultural mistakes. Be respectful. Avoid using employees as interpreters. Use medically competent and fluent interpreters.

How should the nurse do post-mortem care?

Do NOT give the body a full bath (clean visible soil). Raise head of bed to 30 degrees and place palms down to prevent discoloration. Put in dentures (if any). ID the body. Maintain vital organs/skin Integrity. Remove IV/Tubes; replace with Band-Aids unless religious preference is to keep in.

Put protective gear on in this order	Take protective gear off in this order
1st. Wash Hands	1st Gloves
2nd Gown	2nd Googles (if needed)
3rd Mask	3rd Gown
4th Goggles (if needed)	4th Mask
5th Gloves	5th Wash Hands

***When you are putting personal protective equipment (PPE) on, pretend that you are standing with your hands above your head and dress from the bottom up. When you are taking PPE off, take it off alphabetically.

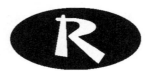

CONSIDER THE CULTURE

People Group	Cultural Considerations
Africans (West, East, North, Central, South)	Subgroups include Angola, Cameroon, Egypt, Ethiopia, Gambia, Ghana, Kenya, Liberia, Nigeria, Namibia, Rwanda, Senegal, Sierra Leone, Sudan, Tanzania, Uganda, Zimbabwe 1. Each ethnic group has a distinct language which will be used whether English is spoken or not. 2. It is socially acceptable for a younger person to call an unrelated older person "sister" or "Auntie." It is not proper to address elders and seniors by their first name. 3. The elders of the family uphold the traditions and cultural norms of the family. 4. Nurses who speak fast will be told to slow down. For example: hurrying behaviors will annoy many Africans as this conveys a lack of concern for adequate care. 5. Africans tend to be more comfortable with narrowed distances and being close together. 6. The nurse should not be surprised to find several family members in the client's room. Let the extra members stay if possible. 7. Prefer to eat their own food instead of hospital food. 8. Will incorporate their faith or religion into the healing process.

African Americans	1. Family is the center of the African American community. The oldest woman in the family may be responsible for medical decisions of the client. 2. Immediate and extended family members may attend medical appointments. Many family members will crowd into the client's room. They should be allowed to stay if there are no disruptions to the delivery of healthcare. 3. Eating "healthy" may feel like giving up a part of their cultural heritage. 4. Patients may feel shame for low health literacy or limited understanding. Silence is a form of respect. 5. Nurses should use the teach back method to evaluate understanding. 6. Singing at the bedside is common. 7. Will incorporate faith or religion into their healing process. It is common for church members to also be considered family. 8. It is best for the nurse to ask the religious affiliation. 9. This group likes to give gifts to say thank you for positive healthcare interactions.
Asian Americans	1. This group highly respects the authority of healthcare workers. 2. Being on time is valued. 3. They may not ask for pain medication or treatments because they do not want to take healthcare workers away from other tasks. 4. Asian Americans may believe health is maintained through a balance of yin (cold) and yang (hot) forces. It is best for the nurse to ask. 6. Do not assume that English is spoken. 7. Asian Americans may not need the same amount of a medication compared to white populations due to slower metabolisms. 8. Inquire about the religious preference for this group.
Caribbeans	Subgroups include: Jamaican, Bahamian, Barbadian, Bermudian, Trinidadian, Belizean, West Indian, Trinidadian and Tobagonian, U.S. Virgin Islander 1. Consider their native islands as "paradise" but leave for opportunities in the States. 2. May believe in myths or health superstitions. 3. They may not take a full course of medication treatment, will report the absence of symptoms or inconvenience of the medication as reasons to stop. 4. Herbal preparations are used in the home to promote healing. 5. Native Caribbean clients tend to self-medicate and exhaust every possible home remedy before seeking medical attention. 6. Religious beliefs and practices may vary. It is best for the nurse to ask. 7. This group does not like to feel rushed during medical visits.
Filipinos	1. They will use the term miracle in relationship to a healing. 2. They like to maintain a principle of balance. 3. They do not want cold drinks in the morning because it will upset the organs. 4. They will be cautious with medical authority. They will be polite but not always trustful. A second opinion is often obtained. 5. Family members may "monitor" medication, other people may be central in the care of client. 6. They may be less likely to seek help for mental illness. 7. They will start greetings by using the term "Sir" or "Ma'am."

Haitians	1. Most believe that not all illnesses can be treated by medical doctors. 2. They believe diseases are often between the head or the heart. 3. The people have a great understanding of herbs and plants that are used for healing. 4. Will prefer to fast rather than eat hospital food. Prefer their own food and may believe American food will make them sicker. 5. Creole is the native language; some also speak French. 6. They are very expressive when in family groups. Being loud is a sign of joy. 7. Health education should be visual and oral to promote increased understanding.

Hispanic/ Latinos	1. There is a wide variety in how pain is handled. Many may turn to religious practices to handle
	   pain.
	2. Delay of treatment often takes place until the illness is severe.
	3. Some may prefer to speak in both English and Spanish at the same time this is common in the
	   Puerto Rican community.
	4. Elderly may prefer to speak in Spanish for important information even if English is understood.
	5. Subgroups of the Hispanic population such as Columbians, Guatemalans, Salvadorans,
	   Peruvians, Nicaraguans, Ecuadorians, Mexicans, Puerto Ricans, Dominicans, and Cubans differ
	   in their lifestyles, health beliefs, and health practices.
	6. Medical decisions will be discussed with the family or community.
	7. Will prefer to eat their own food instead of hospital food.

Indians (South Asia)	Countries include: Bangladesh, Bhutan, India, Maldives, Nepal, Pakistan, Sri Lanka
	1. The concept of purity is important during healthcare practices. Rituals of cleanliness may be practiced each morning.
	2. The nurse should never remove any jewelry the patient is wearing without consent.
	   Jewelry can have religious meaning to the patient.
	3. A vegetarian diet may be expected, some may avoid dairy products.
	4. Ayurvedic medicine and remedies may be used in conjunction with Western medicine.
	5. A same sex healthcare provider should be accommodated.
	6. Women may be considered impure or unclean when menstruating or following childbirth.
	7. The top of the head is considered the most important part of the human body. To touch
	   the head especially on a baby or child is rude.

Religion	**Religious Considerations**
Buddhists	1. They hold to personal insight, do not believe in any kind of deity or God. 2. There is the study of karma, the law of cause and effect. 3. They will prefer to avoid mind-alerting medications while dying. 4. Chanting and prayers are practiced. 5. They usually eat a vegetarian diet. 6. They are encouraged to avoid alcohol, coffee, and tobacco. 7. They do not believe in healing through faith. 8. Medications are acceptable if they do not alter the client's state of mind. 9. There aren't restrictions on autopsy, blood or blood products, organ donations or procedures. 10. They believe in a continuous cycle of life, death, and rebirth.

Islam/ Muslims	1. Believe in one God, Allah. Also study Allah's final prophet Muhammad. 2. Believe in life after death. 3. Will read the Quran. 4. They are required to pray 5 times facing Mecca. Avoid nursing care during prayer time. 5. They wash the face, hands, and feet before prayer. 6. Ramadan is a month long fast of drink, food, and no sexual intercourse during daylight. 7. Pork, shellfish, and alcohol are prohibited. 8. No restrictions on amputations, biopsies, blood or blood products, or medications. 9. Organ donation is acceptable. 10. Healthcare providers are seen as helpers of Allah's will. 11. Abortion is prohibited except in incest, rape or when the mother's life is threatened. 12. Same sex providers are required. 13. Women do not take off their hijab in front of men for any reason. 14. Women are considered impure or unclean when menstruating or following childbirth.
Jehovah's Witness	1. Believe God is the father, Jesus Christ is the son. 2. They do not give gifts on holidays and do not recognize birthdays. 3. Prayer and reading of scriptures are common. They have their own Bible called The New World Translation. 4. Will refuse blood transfusions and blood products as it is against their written scriptures. 5. Abortion is forbidden. 6. An autopsy is acceptable if it is legally required. 7. Believes that after death the beneficiaries of Christ will be resurrected with healthy bodies.
Orthodox Jewish	1. Believes in one all-powerful God who created the universe. 2. Will read the Torah, it is divine and unalterable. 3. Daily prayers are practiced. 4. Yom Kippur: This is a religious fast (no eating or drinking), Day of Atonement. 5. The religious leader is called a rabbi, not a priest. 6. Sabbath (Saturday) is observed as a holy day of rest. 7. May request kosher-certified foods. 8. No pork, shellfish, or unclean meats are consumed in the diet. 9. Autopsy and organ donation are acceptable. 10. The savings of amputated limbs may be required to have a burial service for the limb. 11. There is a belief in life after death. 12. Burial after death is required as soon as possible.
Protestants	1. Includes Amish, Baptists, Christians, Lutherans, Episcopalians, Methodists, Mennonites, Presbyterian, United Church of Christ, Pentecostals, many more. 2. Community worship is important. 3. There is an emphasis on reading the Holy Bible. 4. They believe Jesus is the son of God and Jesus's name is above all names. 5. 2 sacraments that are performed: Baptism and Communion 6. Autopsy and organ donation are acceptable. 7. No diet restrictions are required. The nurse should ask the individual. 8. Daily praying may be performed, will also call for Pastors and others to pray. 9. The cross is a religious symbol. 10. Blood and blood products are an individual's choice. 11. No clinical issues that restrict healthcare. 12. Amish *do not eat pork or shellfish, do not practice birth control, and most reject health insurance. They also prefer midwives and doctors who understand their culture.

Roman Catholicism	1. The largest Christian church, that teaches the One, Holy, Apostolic Church founded by Jesus Christ. 2. Autopsy and organ donation are acceptable. 3. Life after death is a belief. 4. Sacrament of the anointing of the sick is important possibly the Last Rites. 5. Patients may avoid meat on Fridays especially during Lent. 6. No general dietary restrictions. 7. Blood and blood products are acceptable. 8. Attendance at Sunday Mass is an obligation. 9. The cross, candles, holy water, and rosary beads are symbols used for prayer. 10. Only natural birth control is recommended. Abortion is prohibited. 11. If an infant is dying, a baptism is required. 12. May pray to saints especially Mary, the mother of Jesus and other patron saints of health.
Seventh-Day Adventist	1. A protestant Christian that observes Sabbath (Saturday), as a holy day of rest. 2. The religion also emphasizes the imminent second coming of Jesus Christ. 3. Believes the body is the temple of God and must be kept holy. 4. Consuming alcohol, coffee, and tea may be refrained by most. 5. A vegetarian diet is emphasized, some may practice fasting. 6. There is an emphasis on healing with therapeutic diets. 7. No restrictions on blood or blood products. 8. Physicians and chaplains are inseparable. 9. Daily prayers may be performed. 10. Abortion is discouraged. 11. Birth control is acceptable. 12. No infant baptism when death is imminent. 13. An ill person may be anointed with oil and Elders may pray over them.
Spirituality-Hawaiian	1. The teachings reflect the daily practices of oneness and self-greatness, known loosely as the "aloha spirit." 2. There is a sense of connection to all those who have departed from the physical world. 3. There is no belief in a final death just a human changing to the spirit form. 4. Aumakua are family guardians and are respected. 5. The body is treated with respect, funerals are not attended by pregnant women. 6. Fasting is a regular practice. 7. No dietary restrictions. 8. Health is considered the connection between mind, body, and spirit. 9. Silence may be used to promote healing. 10. A newborn baby's name may be delayed due to visions or dreams. 11. Chanting is done for value and respect. 12. Religious history and traditions are handed down through stories.
Spirituality-Native American	1. The Native American's religious and spiritual practices can vary widely. 2. They may use God and Creator interchangeably. 3. They believe in connectedness in all natural things (life, land, and Mother Earth). 4. Prayers often include the use of sacred objects. 5. After death the body is prepared for burial by the family or the tribe. 6. Ill health may be a failure to live in harmony with nature. 7. Elders or a medicine person may lead in healing. 8. A medicine bag is a leather pouch worn around the neck that should not be touched by the nurse. 9. There are no written scriptures.

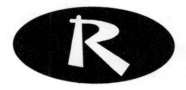

PHARMACOLOGY SECTION

Featuring:

The Top 200 Drugs You Must Know for NCLEX Next Gen!

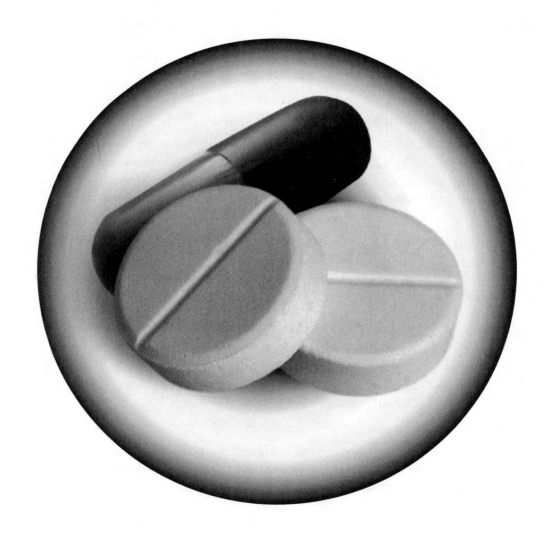

Allergy Medications

Drug	Diphenhydramine
Routes	PO, IV, IM
Use	<ul><li>Antihistamine</li><li>Sedative</li><li>Prevention of an allergic response</li><li>Prevention of nausea and vomiting</li></ul> Doctor will prescribe this medication to patients if they need to take a medication to which they are allergic (for example, blood or IV contrast before a CT). Some travel nurses take this to sleep on planes.

Can. Will. Must. Pass NCLEX!

Drug	Cetirizine -Fexofenadine -Loratadine
Route	PO
Use	<ul><li>Antihistamine</li><li>Common colds</li><li>Rhinitis</li></ul>
NCLEX Tips	This will cause dry mouth & TACHYCARDIA. Patients should take this medication on an empty stomach. It will also cause drowsiness. Do not give to breastfeeding women.

You Didn't Come This Far to Leave Without a Nursing License!

Drug	Beclomethas<u>one</u>	Fluticas<u>one</u>	Mometas<u>one</u>	Triamcinol<u>one</u>
Route	Nasal Sprays			
Use	<ul><li>Rhinitis</li><li>Chronic asthma</li></ul>			
NCLEX Tips	All of these can cause oral fungal infections, hoarseness, and epistaxis. The nurse should teach patients to rinse mouth after each use & seek regular peak flow monitoring.			

Analgesics

Non-opioid Type

Drug	Acetaminophen	Naproxen	NSAIDs	Aspirin (ASA)
Uses		This medication treats mild to moderate pain, fever, arthritis.		
Safety Point	Acetylcysteine is the antidote for an overdose.	Increased risk for heart attack and stroke	These two medications have an anti-platelet use also ototoxicity risk is present. Reye's syndrome can occur if ASA is used for viral infections.	
NCLEX Tips	Do not give to clients with liver failure.	These can cause GI bleeding. Stop taking a week before surgery. Do not administer with anticoagulants. Take this medication with food.		

Don't talk about it, be about it! And now it's time to work!

Opioid / Narcotic Type

Drug	Morphine	Hydromorphone	Codeine	Meperidine hcl	Oxycodone
NCLEX Tips	Will cause respiratory depression. Don't give if breaths are under 10. Monitor for constipation. Addiction may occur with long term use. Take with food to prevent nausea.				
Safety Point	Hydromorphone is many more times stronger than morphine. Codeine is used as cough suppressant. Meperidine increases intracranial pressure do not give for ICP. Do not give oxycodone to clients allergic to acetaminophen.				

Antibiotics

Antibiotics	Examples	How they help	How they harm
Aminoglycosides	Streptomycin Azithromycin Gentamycin *Vancomycin is a macrolide but has the same side effects.	Meningitis Infective endocarditis Septicemia C-difficile	Ototoxicity and nephrotoxicity risk Effects on hearing: ringing and dizziness. Do not give during pregnancy. Draw a peak & trough (blood test). Draw the peak 30 minutes after giving the medication if the route was IV. Draw the peak 1 hour after if the route was PO. Draw the trough 30 minutes before final dose. *The antidote is calcium gluconate.*
Penicillin (PCN)	Penicillin Amoxicillin Ampicillin	Gonorrhea Pneumonia UTI	First ask about a history of allergies. DO NOT GIVE IF ANY reaction has occurred in the past. Safe for pregnant or breastfeeding women. The first time a client takes PCN, stay with them for the first 15 minutes. *Epinephrine is the antidote for an allergic reaction.* Educate the client to take the medication for the full prescribed length of time.
Tetracyclines	Doxycycline Demecyclines Minocycline	UTI Pneumonia Gonorrhea Syphilis May be given if the patient is allergic to PCN.	Can cause phototoxicity, nephrotoxicity, and hepatotoxicity. Keep out of direct sunlight, monitor liver enzymes, kidney function, labs and urine output. Do not give if patient is pregnant or breastfeeding. Do not give with cow's milk. Do not give to children under 8 years old; will cause teeth to turn black. Give this medication with a straw ☺ Avoid giving with Lasix.
Cephalosporins	Cefazolin Cephalexin	UTI, Pneumonia, Gonorrhea Do not give if allergic to PCN!	Side Effects: Remember that cephalosporins will leave you HAIRY. **H**-yperglycemic **A**-naphylatic shock (if allergic) **I**-nsufficient platelets (thrombocytopenia) **R**-enal problems (nephrotoxic) **Y**-ellow poop (diarrhea) *Epinephrine is the antidote.*
Ciprofloxacin	Ciprofloxacin	Bacterial infections Respiratory anthrax Urinary tract infections	Photosensitivity GI distress (nausea, vomiting, diarrhea) With this medication a false positive on a urine drug screen will show for opiates. In children there is a concern this drug may cause arthrotoxicity.

Anti-Coagulants

	Heparin	Warfarin
Onset	Less than one hour	4-10 days
Short term or Long term	Short term	Long term
Routes	IV or SQ	PO only
Labs to watch	PTT PTT should be 1.5-2.5 times the control	INR or PT INR should be 2-3.
Antidote	Protamine sulfate	Vitamin K
Pregnancy Safe	Yes, you can give	No, don't give, there is a baby in there!
Will this medication break down a clot?	No	No
Potential complications of the drug therapy	Heparin induced thrombocytopenia (HIT)	Coumadin induced necrosis

1. Be careful; some herbal medications can interfere with anticoagulants.
2. Tell patients to stop taking two weeks before surgery.
3. Frequent blood draws will be needed during the beginning of treatment.

	Enoxaparin
Indication	Prevent deep vein thromboses (DVT)
Route	Subcutaneous injection or IV (less common)
Assessment	Medication should be clear with no particles or discoloration before injecting. Monitor for signs of bleeding.
Contraindications	Do not give if client has a history of heparin-induced thrombocytopenia. Patients should stop taking 24 hours before surgery. Do not administer with other blood thinners.
ReMar Notes	This is considered a *Low Molecular Weight Heparin (LMWH)* <u>The benefits of LMWH over Heparin:</u> Once daily injections. No lab monitoring. This can be prescribed as outpatient therapy.

Anti-Convulsants

Drug	Phenobarbital	Phenytoin	Valproic acid	Gabapentin
NCLEX Tips	Decreases BP and RESPIRATIONS Vitamin D supplement may be needed.	Do not give with food, do not take with oral birth control pills.	Hepatotoxic agent Watch for abdominal cramping. May cause suicidal thoughts.	May cause memory problems. Do administer with antacids. Will help with symptoms of restless leg syndrome.

In general, all anti-convulsants:

- Can become toxic in the body system or cause dependency issues.
- Cause drowsiness.
- Should not be taken with antacids, which will decrease absorption.
- Can elevate the blood glucose levels.
- May change the urine to a light rust color, but it is not dangerous to the client.
- Will still allow the client to have a seizure despite being on medication.
- The client should be educated to wear their medical ID bracelet at all times.
- Do not give any of these medications before electroconvulsive therapy.

Safety Point	***If the client is on an anti-convulsant, initiate seizure precautions!**

Antidotes

Medication	Antidotes [5]
Magnesium Sulfate	Calcium Gluconate
Acetaminophen	N-acetylcysteine (oral form)
Insulin	Glucagon
Morphine (other narcotics)	Naloxone
High potassium (k+)	Insulin (IV), Sodium polystyrene sulfonate
Benzodiazepines	Flumazenil
Methotrexate	Leucovorin

Antineoplastics

Drug	Cisplatin	Cyclophosphamide	Methotrexate	Tamoxifen
NCLEX Tips	May cause tinnitus, blurry vision, and fever. Electrolyte imbalances will occur • Hypokalemia • Hypocalcemia • Hypomagnesemia • Hypophosphatemia	Rinse mouth to prevent stomatitis. May cause sterility.	May cause thrombocytopenia. May cause toxicity. The antidote is leucovorin.	Affects women: causes hot flashes, irregular menstruation, vaginal bleeding & discharge.
	Patients need to increase fluids to 2-3 liters per day.			

In general, antineoplastics:

- A client's weight should be taken the day of medication administration.

- Clients should avoid vaccinations during therapy.

- Medications can cause an increase in uric acid (hyperuricemia).

- Some clients will be given blood thinners with cancer medications to increase effectiveness.

- Use bleeding precautions.

- Special handling may be required (cytotoxic).

  May cause future birth defects, no pregnant or breastfeeding nurses to care for client.

  Gowns, gloves, face protection if administering a liquid.

  Gloves (1-pair) if administering a solid.

  If applying creams to the patient the nurse should wear two pairs of gloves.

- Extravasation may occur at IV site.

  1st priority: stop infusion, keep the IV catheter in place.

  2nd priority: Notify primary health care provider.

Anti-Parkinson's

Drugs	Benztropine	Carbidopa/Levodopa	Selegiline
Mechanism of action	Anticholinergic	Increases dopamine	MAO inhibitor
NCLEX Tips	Do not administer with antihistamines. May cause fever. May help with extrapyramidal symptoms caused by psychiatric medications.	Eat a low protein diet as protein interferes with this medication. Can cause false positive ketones in the urine. Can cause hemolytic anemia.	May cause sexual dysfunction. Avoid food high in tyramine. The client should not stop taking this medication abruptly.

Side Effects of Anti-Parkinson medications

A - Altered vital signs, Avoid sudden movements.
B - Blurry vision
C - Constipation, confusion
D - Dry mouth, dizziness

- Teach clients to self-monitor for improvement of Parkinson's symptoms.
- Tell clients do not stop this medication abruptly.

Beta Blockers

Ending	"olol"		
Examples	metoprolol, atenolol,		
Indication	Hypertension, angina, treatment of myocardial infarction		
Action	Blocks Epinephrine and norepinephrine from binding to beta receptors on the nerves		
Effects	Decreases BP, Pulse, Increases Heart CONTRACTILITY force		
Contraindications	Hold if the heart rate is less than 60. Beta blockers may block the signs of low blood sugar. They should be used in caution in diabetic patients. Beta blockers can cause an increase in cholesterol. Beta blockers can also make asthma and COPD worse.		
Antidote	Glucagon		

*Generic names with a different ending instead of "olol" labetalol carvedilol

Clinical Priorities	1. Teach patient do not stop taking beta blockers abruptly.
	2. Teach the client to take this medication with meals and change positions slowly.
	3. Monitor the blood glucose levels in patients with diabetes taking a beta blocker.
	4. The nurse should monitor blood pressure, heart rate, and ALT, AST, BUN, Creatinine.

Cardiac Medications

Medication Names	Dopamine	Epinephrine	Phenylephrine	Norepinephrine
Administration Notes	Onset 5 minutes	Onset Immediate	Onset Immediate	Onset 15-20 minutes
Clinical Use	Heart failure Will increase urine output in clients with renal failure.	Cardiac Arrest Anaphylactic Shock	Vasodilatory Shock Hemorrhagic Shock Will raise blood pressure but not heart rate.	Septic Shock Can cause mottling

Drugs	Angiotensin-Converting Enzyme (ACE) Inhibitors	Angiotensin Receptor Blockers (ARBS)	Calcium Channel Blockers (CCB)	Thiazide Diuretics
Generic Names	Drugs that end in "pril" Lisinopril Captopril Enalapril	Drugs that end in "sartan" Losartan Valsartan	Amlodipine Nifedipine Verapamil Diltiazem	Drugs that end in "thiazide" Hydrochlorothiazide Chlorothiazide
Action	Block the enzyme that converts angiotensin 1 into angiotensin 2 – (a super-powerful vasoconstrictor that will increase the BP.) Angiotensin 2 also causes the secretion of an additional blood pressure elevating hormone in the adrenal glands called aldosterone.)	Blocks the effects of angiotensin 2 at the receptor sites.	Stops calcium from entering the myocardium muscles which promotes vasodilation.	Increases the release of sodium and potassium which results in *hypokalemia.*
Clinical Priorities	Avoid in African American patients due to increased risk of angioedema. Listen for a "dry, hacking, cough. Do not give if the patient has a history of angioedema or renal impairment. Avoid during pregnancy. Can increase potassium levels.	ARBS may raise potassium levels. Give at bedtime to better control blood pressure. Avoid grapefruit juice with losartan.	Nifedipine ER is safe to give during pregnancy. Do not give in clients with heart block. Do not give with grapefruit juice.	Avoid in clients who have a sulfa allergy. Causes photosensitivity. Administer in the morning to prevent nocturia. Decreases the effectiveness of antidiabetic medications. Avoid giving with lithium.

Cardiac Medications

Name	Digoxin
Action	Nobody really knows exactly how digoxin
Effects	Slows down the heart rate. Increases BP and tissue perfusion.
Clinical Priorities	Always take an apical pulse hold if HR is less than 60 in adults and less than 100 in infants. Therapeutic level is 1-2. If greater than 2, client is digoxin toxic. Signs of digoxin toxicity: The client will see yellow spots, nausea, vomiting, and abdominal pain. WARNING the sign of toxicity in infants and children is bradycardia. Nurses must monitor potassium levels. A low potassium level can increase the risk of digoxin toxicity. If client becomes toxic, give activated charcoal or digoxin immune fab.

Name	Nitroglycerin
Action	It is a vasodilator given to reduce preload and afterload of the heart
Effects	It lowers blood pressure and increases the oxygenation of tissues
Contraindications	Do not take with sildenafil citrate. A client can take one or the other, but never both as it causes severe hypotension! When nitro SL, a nurse can give only up to three tablets over 15 minutes. Give one tablet every five minutes. Call emergency medical services after second tablet of nitroglycerin is given. Do NOT eat or drink while taking it. If giving nitroglycerin via a patch, never place over a pacemaker and remove the patch before client goes into MRI. If the MD orders nitro IV, place on an infusion pump always!

Diuretics

Type	Examples	NCLEX Tips
Carbonic Anhydrase Inhibitors	Acetazolamide	This medication is best for open angle glaucoma ocular pressure control.
Loop	Furosemide Bumetanide	This is the fastest acting. It can be given PO or IV. Watch for a decreased potassium level. May cause ototoxicity (the chance will increase when given with an Aminoglycoside). Used for acute edema (pulmonary or CHF).
Osmotic	Mannitol	Used to get rid of water instead of sodium. Best for increased intracranial pressure.
Potassium-sparing	Spironolactone	Used orally, not as powerful as loop diuretics. Watch for an increase in potassium level. Do not give to patients with diabetes mellitus. Best diuretic for hyperaldosteronism. This may cause agranulocytosis.
Thiazide	Hydrochlorothiazide	Used for chronic hypertension. This is a slow acting diuretic. Increases the toxicity effect in heart medications such as quinidine and digoxin. This decreases the effectiveness of antidiabetic agents.

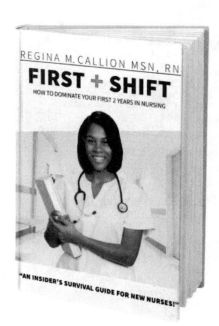

GI Medications

Stops Nausea & Vomiting

Drug	Client Teaching
Ondansetron	Give 30-minutes before chemo or one-hour before radiation. May cause headache. Do not give oral tablets to clients with phenylketonuria because they contain aspartame which forms phenylalanine.
Promethazine	*Psychiatric medication that can be used for nausea. May cause false positive pregnancy test.
Meclizine	Used for motion sickness or dizziness. Take 1-hour before traveling.

Stops Diarrhea

Drug	Client Teaching
Loperamide	Watch for constipation; this may also cause rebound constipation. Be cautious if giving to clients with C-difficile or infectious diarrhea. Take 30-minutes before a meal.

Starts Diarrhea

Drug	Client Teaching
Lactulose	This is a PO laxative given to reduce **ammonia** levels (encephalopathy); works within 15-minutes. Contains sugars (lactose). Use with caution in clients with diabetes.
Polystyrene Sulfonate	This is a rectal or PO laxative given to reduce **potassium** levels; works within 15-minutes. Do not give if client has paralytic issues.
Psyllium	This is a dietary fiber to cause fecal matter to expand and increase bowel movements. Mix with 8 oz. of water
Docusate Sodium	*Stool softener; takes several days to work. Teach the clients do not split the pills or chew them.
Magnesium Hydroxide Salts	*Stool softener salts that cause stool to expand in intestine.
General Teaching for all medications in this group	Do not to patients with unknown abdominal pain.

Drug	Examples	Teaching
Antacids	Calcium carbonate	Give 1-hour after meals with a full glass of water. Can cause hypercalcemia. Do not give with antibiotics.
Histamine 2 blocker (H2 blockers)	Famotidine Cimetidine	Used to prevent ulcers and reduces stomach acid. Give with or before meals.
Proton pump inhibitors	Omeprazole, Pantoprazole	Take 60 minutes before meals. Do not chew. May cause liver failure.
Simethicone	Simethicone	Chew tablets. Take after meals.

Protects the Mucosal Lining of the Stomach

Drug	Teaching
Sucralfate	Give PO and take on an empty stomach. Do not crush or chew. May cause hyperglycemia. Do not give with warfarin or phenytoin.

Insulins

Types	Generic Name	Onset	Peak	Duration
Rapid Acting Used in wearable insulin pumps	**Insulin Aspart Insulin lispro** Administer with meals. Do not mix with other insulins.	Less than 15-minutes	1-hour	3-hours
Short Acting "clear"	**Regular** The only insulin that can be given IV route.	1-hour	2-hours	4-hours
Intermediate "cloudy"	NPH	4-hours	8-hours	12-hours
Long Acting Cannot mix this insulin with any of the others.	**Insulin determir Insulin glargine**	Slow absorption	No peak	24-hours Give same time daily.
Pre-Mixed Insulin 70/30	Humulin 70/30 70% is NPH / 30% is Regular	30-minutes	2-hours	16 hours

Oral Antidiabetic Agents

General Client Teaching:

These medications act on the pancreas to stimulate insulin production.
These medications are for diabetes mellitus 2 only.
These medications must be taken with meals.

Glucophage	Glipizide Glyburide	Rosiglitazone Maleate	Exenatide
Do not give before or 48-hours after an intravenous pyelogram (IVP) together they can cause kidney damage.	Administer in the morning. May drop blood glucose levels quickly. Have a snack available. This medication can cause jaundice.	Can cause jaundice. May decrease the effectiveness of oral contraceptives.	*This is a subcutaneous injectable medication May cause GI distress. Not recommended for clients also taking insulin.

Client Teaching:

Contraindicated medications to give with oral antidiabetic agents

1. Warfarin
2. Oral contraceptives
3. Corticosteroids

* My first paycheck as a nurse, I made a whopping $2,700.00! Whoo-hoo ☺

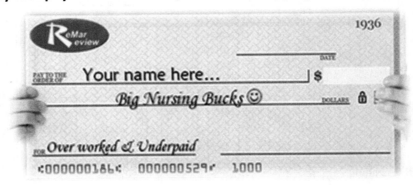

Natural Alternatives

Herbal	Action	Client Teaching
St. John's Wort	Treats depression/anxiety	Interacts with SSRIs Can cause sun sensitivity. Decreases the effect of digoxin.
Garlic	Lowers BP/cholesterol	1 clove equals 4 grams of garlic. Interacts with warfarin and aspirin
Ginkgo Biloba	Improves memory	Thins the blood. Do not take with warfarin and aspirin. Can interfere with seizure medication
Ginseng	Increased physical stamina. Reduces tinnitus and ringing in the ears.	Can cause hypertension when mixed with caffeine. Increases risk for bleeding.
Echinacea	Prevents cold and flu has an immune-boosting function	Can cause liver toxicity in renal patients, not effective with HIV.
Ginger	Relieves nausea and vomiting	Do not take if there is a history of DVT Interacts with blood thinners.
Black Cohosh	Treats menopausal symptoms	Can be used to treat hot flashes. Contraindicated in pregnancy it will cause premature labor.
Kava Kava	Treats insomnia, muscle pain	Will cause a decrease in the effectiveness of Parkinson's disease medications. Can increase the risk of suicide in clients with depression.
Saw Palmetto	Used for prostate health	Reduces the absorption of iron. *Risk for false positive prostate specific antigen test. Will have a diuretic effect.

General client teaching:

All herbal medications that start with the letter G thin the blood; do not give with warfarin, aspirin, or heparin.

All herbal medications are contraindicated during pregnancy and lactation.

Herbal medications should be stopped 2-weeks before surgery due to the possible interaction with anesthesia.

What's harder...studying for NCLEX or getting out of bed at 5:00 a.m. for clinicals?

109

Maternity

Medication that STARTS Contractions	Oxytocin
	*Assess character, frequency, and duration of uterine contractions. Stop oxytocin when contractions are 2 minutes apart and lasts more than 60 seconds. Monitor fetal heart rate every 15 minutes. This medication releases milk in pregnant women. This medication is IV piggybacked into a main IV line. *This medication has an antidiuretic effect and can cause water intoxication in the patient. (Fluid overload complications)

Medication that STOPS Contractions	Terbutaline Sulfate & Ritodrine
NCLEX Tips	Causes tachycardia in mother & baby. Decreases potassium levels.

Medication that reduces pain	*Butorphanol
NCLEX Tips	Binds to opiate receptors to reduce labor pain. Side effects include: drowsiness, dizziness, confusion, respiratory depression, nausea, vomiting, bradycardia, and hypotension. (These are typical side effects of opioid analgesics.) This is contraindicated in clients with renal complications and history of opioid dependency.

Lower Blood Pressure in Pre-eclampsia	Magnesium sulfate
NCLEX Tips	This medication decreases respirations, reflexes, and urine output. An indwelling catheter may be needed to monitor urine output. The nurse should monitor reflexes and respirations as well. The antidote for an increased magnesium sulfate level is calcium gluconate.

Stops Post-Partum Hemorrhage/Bleeding	Methergine
NCLEX Tips	Prevents post-partum/post abortion bleeding. Given as an IM injection. Can cause severe hypertensive crisis. Do not give before delivery of the placenta. *Side effects: dizziness, headache, tinnitus, cardiac palpations, *ergotism (cold fingers & toes which can also lead to gangrene) Can cause severe hypertensive crisis. Smoking should be avoided as it increases vasoconstriction. Drinking grapefruit juice can increase medication levels. Teach the client not to breastfeed for at least 12 hours after using this medication. Beta blockers & dopamine may increase the medication levels.

Increases Fetal Lung Maturity	Betamethasone
NCLEX Tips	Administered antenatally. *Indication: Given at 34-36 weeks' gestation if imminent birth to increase fetal lung maturation Route: IM Dose: Two 12 mg doses 24 hours apart Side effects are hypertension, pruritus, and hyperglycemia.

Take the FINAL Step with the NCLEX-V2!

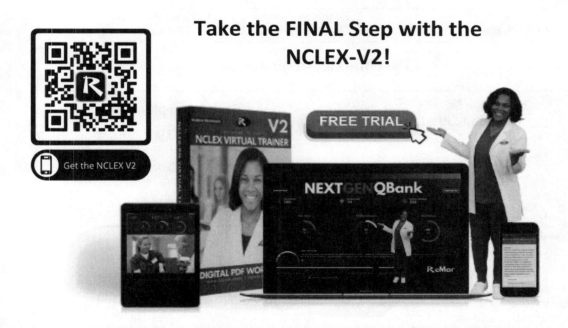

Respiratory Medications

Drugs	Theophylline Aminophylline	Albuterol	Montelukast	Fluticasone propionate
Class	Bronchodilator			
NCLEX Tips	Will cause tachycardia. Monitor for toxicity. Normal levels are 10-20. Patients should avoid caffeine in the diet.	Used for acute or severe asthma attacks. Will cause tachycardia. May cause tremors.	Do not give for severe asthma attacks. This medication takes a long time to work. Administer in the evening.	Do not give for severe asthma attacks. After opening, the diskus is good for one month. Teach the patient to never exhale into the diskus.

Always administer bronchodilators first before you give steroids when doing breathing treatments. Remember that with aerosol therapy the amount of the medication the client receives cannot be measured. However, aerosols work the fastest by going straight to the lungs.

Drug	Beclomethasone
Class of drug	Corticosteroid
NCLEX tips	Used for chronic asthma. Helps produce surfactant, rinse mouth after administration

Drugs	Guaifenesin
Class of drug	Expectorant
NCLEX tips	Take this medication with a full glass of water. Increased fluid is needed to loosen the secretions.

Psychiatric Medications

<u>**Classification**</u> **Anti-anxiety**	**Benzodiazepines** Medications that end in – ZEPAM Alprazolam Clona<u>zepam</u> Dia<u>zepam</u> Lora<u>zepam</u> Tema<u>zepam</u>
Side effects Side effects are ABCDS A-Altered vital signs (bradycardia, low BP) B-Blurry vision C-Constipation, confusion D-Dry mouth, dizziness S-Stasis of urine, sedation	**NCLEX Tips** Very addictive. Short-term use only. Do not stop taking abruptly. Watch for respiratory depression.
If client overdoses on benzodiazepines administer flumazenil.	

It is often the small steps not the giant leaps that bring about lasting change.

Non-benzodiazepines	
These medications also work on anxiety	
Buspirone	**Zolpidem**
Use: Obsessive Compulsive Disorder Post-Traumatic Stress Disorder This medication has a lower sedative effect than a benzodiazepine. This medication should not be taken with grapefruit juice.	Use: Insomnia This medication should be administered immediately before sleep. Headaches are a reported side effect. Clients can become psychologically dependent. Sleep walking is common.

Classification **Anti-depressants**	**Selective Serotonin Reuptake Inhibitors (SSRI)** Fluoxetine-administer in the morning. Citalopram Sertraline
Side effects Agitation, anorexia Blurred vision Constipation Dry mouth Sleep disturbances	**NCLEX Tips** This causes suicidal ideation. May take 4-6 weeks to work. Do not give with disulfiram. Clients should not drink alcohol with this medication. Never administer an SSRI and a MAOI together.

Psychiatric Medications

Classification **Anti-depressants**	**Monoamine Oxidase Inhibitors (MAOI)** Isocarboxazid, Phenelzine, Tranylcypromine
Side Effects Anorexia Blurred vision Constipation Dry mouth Excessive sweating Muscle rigidity	Never give MAOIs with SSRIs. This medication takes four to six weeks to work. Know dietary restrictions; your client will not be allowed to eat anything with tyramine in it. Tyramine and taking an MAOI together can cause severe hypertension.

Tyramine-Restricted Diet

The food clients CAN NOT have:

Meats	No organ or preserved. No bacon, sausage, bologna, peperoni, salami, luncheon meat with nitrates
Grains	No grains with active yeast
Vegetables	No BAR (Bananas, Avocados, or Raisins)
Fruits	No BAR again
Dairy	No cheese except cottage, No yogurt
Sweets/Oils	No coffee, tea, or chocolate
Soy Products	No soy sauce, tofu, or teriyaki
Nuts & Seeds	No nuts, peanut butter, or pumpkin seeds

The food clients CAN have:

1. Decaffeinated coffee
2. Fruit juices
3. Club soda
4. All types of pastas
5. All cooked and dry cereals.

Psychiatric Medications

Anti-Psychotics	
Typical Medications	Thorazine Compazine Stelazine Promethazine Haloperidol Chlorpromazine
Routes	PO, IV, IM (IM route lasts the longest)
Indication	Positive Psychotic Symptoms: Delusions Hallucinations Neologisms
Side Effects	Extrapyramidal Symptoms Agitation Blurred vision Constipation Difficulty urinating Dry mouth, Drowsiness Erectile dysfunction *Benztropine can be given to reduce extrapyramidal side effects
Adverse Effects	Neuroleptic Malignant Syndrome

Anti-Psychotics	
Atypical Medications	Clozapine Risperidone Aripriprazole Olanzapine Quetiapine
Routes	PO, IV, IM (IM route lasts the longest)
Indication	Positive Psychotic Symptoms: Delusions Hallucinations Neologisms
Side Effects	Metabolic changes such as: Hyperglycemia Dyslipidemia Weight gain
Adverse Effects	Agranulocytosis

Psssst… Hey, You're Almost There!

Once you've passed Next Gen go to **ReMarNurse.com/PARTY** to share your NCLEX Journey and claim your FREE ReMar Nurse Tee to help us celebrate this accomplishment!

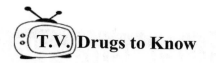

T.V. Drugs to Know

Drug	Indication	Client Teaching
Ibandronate	Postmenopausal Osteoporosis Paget's disease	Bone pain may occur as a side effect. Sit up for 60 minutes after taking. Take on an empty stomach.
Alendronate	Osteoporosis in men and women Paget's disease	Caffeine and orange juice decrease absorption. Sit up for 60 minutes. Take on empty stomach.
Sildenafil/ Tadalafil	Treats pulmonary and arterial hypertension (in women) Erectile dysfunction (in men)	Given 1 to 4 hours before sexual activity. Do not take with nitroglycerin! May cause a sudden drop in BP
Allopurinol	Anti-gout	Can cause kidney stones. Do not eat organ meat, alkaline diet preferred. Make sure to drink eight glasses of water a day to prevent kidney stones.
(Onabotulinumtoxin A)	Temporary muscle relaxant	May cause eyelid to droop. Do not give during pregnancy. Clients with HIV can take.
Clopidogrel	Blood thinner	Need to do platelet count. Excessive bleeding Severe confusion
Bupropion	Smoking cessation Antidepressants Sexual dysfunction in women	Taper off medication May cause insomnia or seizures. Monitor for suicidal thoughts.

Quick Facts Pharmacology Sheet

Medication by Route

Dermal Patch	Nasal Spray	Rectal	Sublingual
• Clonidine • Fentanyl • Nicotine patch • Oxybutynin • Selegiline • Testosterone	• Butorphanol • Fentanyl • Nicotine nasal spray • Cyanocobalamin	• Bisacodyl suppositories • Diazepam suppositories • Ergotamine suppositories • Glycerin suppositories	• Cyanocobalamin • Fentanyl • Nitroglycerin • Zolpidem

Medications That Make Conditions Worse

Allergies	Anxiety	Blood Pressure	Cholesterol
• Eggs: • Propofol • Yellow fever vaccine • Peanut/Soy: • Dimercaprol • Progesterone capsules • Valproic acid • Sulfa: • Acetazolamide • Celecoxib • Glyburide • Sulfamethoxazole-trimethoprim	• Apriprazole • Bupropion • Caffeine • Cocaine • Decongestants • Methamphetamine	• Appetite suppressants • Caffeine • Corticosteroids • Excessive alcohol (1-2 drinks daily) • Herbal medications-ephedra, St. John's Wort • Thyroid hormone	• Atypical antipsychotics • Beta blocker • Isotretinoin
Depression	**Dementia**	**Causes Hyperkalemia**	**Vision Problems**
• Anabolic steroids • Clonidine • Cyclosporine • Indomethacin • Methyldopa	• Benztropine • Antipsychotics • Benzodiazepines • Skeletal muscle relaxants	• Amiloride • Cyclosporine • Heparin • Potassium in TPN • Spironolactone	• Anticholinergics • Ethambutol • Hydroxychloroquine • Isoniazid • Isotretinoin • Tamoxifen

Medications That Change the Color of Sweat, Tears, & Urine

- Levodopa/Carbidopa
- Metronidazole
- Propofol
- Pyrazinamide
- Rifampin

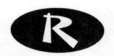

Congratulations on Completing *Quick Facts* for NCLEX®
You're now an official studying member of the ReMar Nurse Family!

Hey ReMar Nurse, I hope that you've enjoyed your studying experience so far. If this is your first time completing Quick Facts I can tell you that most of my students go back over this book two and three times. It was my goal to make this NCLEX study guide very easy to understand. I believe true education should not drain you. It should bring life, hope, and a better outlook for your goals.

As I said before, memorize everything in this book. Most students like to use this book two and three times before testing.

Passing NCLEX is too important to take lightly or leave it up to chance! Out of all the emails and messages that I get from students are the testimonials from ReMar Nurses that were struggling with this exam but someone told them about ReMar! Here's

You didn't come this far to leave without your license!"

"Thank you so much Professor Regina! I passed NCLEX because a friend told me about ReMar. I wasn't sure but I got your review program and did EVERYTHING and I'm so glad I did!"

I want to let you know you're on the right track. Also, I'm super proud that you've completed this book!

For best results we recommend the NCLEX V2 which you can complete in 30 days or less!

Taking the Next Steps on Your Road to NCLEX!

As you can see, *Quick Facts for NCLEX* is the foundation of our comprehensive training but there's so much more content to learn before you're ready to take Next Gen.

I've heard from too many students who have tested MULTIPLE TIMES and I want to help you break that cycle especially if you know you are a difficult tester or have testing anxiety.

I've personally put my best into this training, and I expect nothing less from you!

With the NCLEX V2 you'll have my **Lectures, NGN Question Bank, CAT Assessments,** and **printable Student Workbook for Next Gen!!**

If you're ready to get started today go to ReMarNurse.com and sign up now for the free NCLEX V2 Trial account to begin training today. If you have any questions, send my team an email to Support@ReMarReview.com and my experts will help you get started right away!

Your passion for nursing is a true blessing. Remember that whenever moments of fear, anxiety, or doubt arise. I'm here for you and can't wait to see your testimony on the other side of NCLEX!

Regina M. Callion MSN, RN
www.ReMarNurse.com

Notes

Notes

Notes

Notes

Notes